CREATIVE
FIRST AID

We dedicate this book to wonky clouds, to birdsong, wigs, coloured pencils and pineapple-shaped sunglasses, and to children, the teachers of creativity. Thanks for all the glimmers!

THE SCIENCE + JOY OF CREATIVITY
FOR MENTAL HEALTH

CREATIVE FIRST AID

Caitlin Marshall + Lizzie Rose

murdoch books
Sydney | London

Contents

Creativity lives within all of us. It's part of being a human, and always has been, therefore every one of us is creative. Like a muscle, creativity can grow stronger the more we use it, so this is your invitation to gently begin flexing your imagination and explore this for yourself. Finding our way to this innate part of ourselves can be challenging, exciting, surprising and unfamiliar. Ultimately, it can be life-changing.

This book is a reminder that you are creative and that your creativity is an extremely useful tool with which to navigate the trickiness of life. It is an invitation to begin or continue a conscious practice of applying creativity to yourself (self-care), to others (community care) and to the environment (care for the planet), as a form of vital first aid.

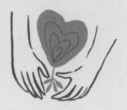

INTRODUCTION

Our story

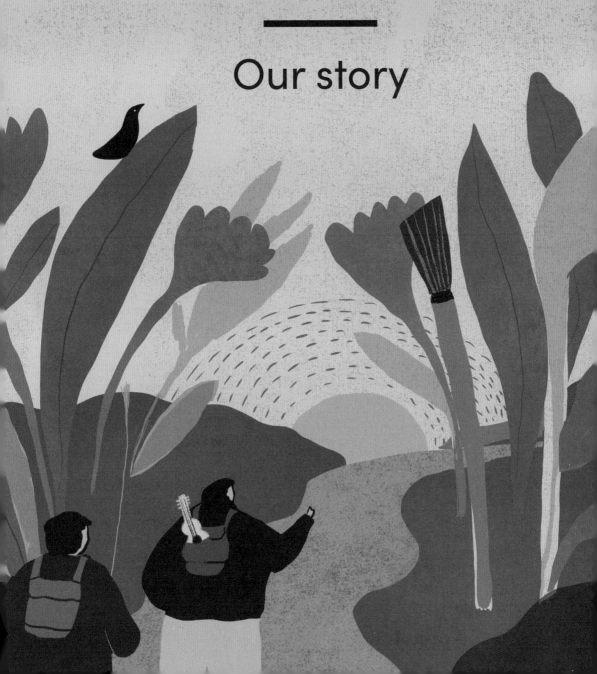

Hello!

Welcome. Have a seat. Or stand, if that's more comfy. Or lie on the floor, even. Comfort is important.

This is a book about mental health. It's also about creativity. We're going to show you how we have helped people recover from trauma using creative first aid. We tell you their stories, show you the evidence, and give you the tools to try this for yourself – tools like self-compassion and charcoal pencils.

We show you how 'making' can shift your mood, and shape your nervous system. MakeShift was founded to prescribe creative practice as a pathway for people to connect to themselves, to others and to the planet.

Our prescriptions offer relief and recovery from trauma, but also from anxiety, depression, overwhelm, illness, isolation – common experiences so many of us live with. Like Margaret, who was over 80 when we met her in a tiny wooden hall in regional NSW. She was there with 12 others who had gathered to work with us to process disaster trauma through drawing as creative first aid. Blank pages quickly filled with portraits, and a steady eruption of laughter was passed around. Margaret, later, her eyes full of tears, spoke of the fires that had ripped through her community, and of how she nearly lost her house. This devastation led to deep disconnection, but she described this small moment of delight in the hall as drawing breath, likening it to coming up for air. With the grace of a deep rest, she said, 'I can breathe again.'

We've learnt firsthand that every single person has innate creativity and, it turns out, using it is good for us.

Why we wrote this book

MakeShift is part of a global movement called Social and Creative Prescribing, which is the intentional use of fun, recreational, creative and social activities to enable shifts towards a healthy, connected, empowered life. This approach is not a new idea. Creativity is an act of joining dots, or making something that wasn't there before. It's a practice that harnesses curiosity, playfulness and experimentation. Prescribed creativity, or creative first aid, as we call it, adds in self-compassion and safekeeping and is sensitive to the trauma and challenges that many people are navigating every day.

Applying creative first aid can be game-changing for our nervous system, the intricate and complex network that comprises our brain, spinal cord and nerves. The nervous system controls most of what we do. It influences our breathing and what we think and feel. It is also the major navigator of how we respond to threat and joy. Understanding how your nervous system works can become a powerful tool in triaging stress, fear and distress.

When we work with our bodies to constantly fine-tune ourselves towards a balanced state of being, a little like a violin that responds to climatic changes and requires regular fine-tuning, it is called *nervous system regulation*. Connecting with our own creativity influences the way we feel about ourselves and the world, and the stories we tell about who we are.

This book makes the case for engaging with your own innate creativity. Firstly, because many people don't believe they are creative at all. Not true! And secondly, while physical exercise has triumphed as a universally accepted activity to improve many things, including our health and wellbeing, creativity has languished as a luxury for a select few. There are strange, unspoken rules about who is allowed to be creative, leaving everyone else to close the door to these practices for most of their adult lives. This is a tragedy, and we are going to show you why.

We also want to broaden the conversation and search for answers that lie beyond the medical model of health and wellbeing. We are zooming out and asking the big questions: what is mental health and what do we need to make sure we are taking care of ourselves? What kind of solutions are we throwing at it, and are these the right ones?

Until prescribing creativity as a mode of health treatment is mainstream, we can start using it ourselves. With permission, self-compassion, curiosity and a little guidance, we can playfully explore our own creativity to develop a trusty toolkit of strategies that are free, accessible and available anytime.

The origins of MakeShift

We met in 2007 at an informal singing group and instantly hit it off. That midwinter evening about half a dozen of us had gathered in someone's garage to ditch the small talk for a cappella. Over the next decade we practised our vocal warm-ups, attempted harmonies and shared melodies, holding space for our voices. These weekly sessions got us all through the big, messy parts of life: birth, death, illness, career changes and the complex range of emotions that mark middle age.

In the beginning, the singing felt like a bit of an experiment. We weren't professionals, we were just trying stuff out. But the more we sang, the more comfortable we got with being out of tune. Eventually, we got pretty good, but that wasn't really the point. The point was how it made us feel. The zing on the back of your neck when you find harmony, and the buzz in your fingertips when a group of voices comes together in unison – there's nothing else like it. A moment of pure joy.

Recreating the experience we'd had in our singing group became the driving force behind MakeShift, as we shared the same core belief that all humans have a deep need for fun. Separately, in our professional experiences so far – working in community development, supporting survivors of violence, and providing sustainability education around climate change – joy and play had felt very far away, and we both felt instinctively that this was a gap that needed to be filled.

MakeShift was founded in 2013 in our local community of Wollongong, on the South Coast of New South Wales, in Lizzie's lounge room. We have always worked on Dharawal Country, whose original custodians, the Wodi Wodi people, hold a rich history of creative practices such as weaving and painting as ways of making records, connections, community and also practical, useful things. These creative forms are still being practised today.

In the beginning, MakeShift was a grassroots skill exchange platform. We ran workshops in backyards, small halls, art galleries and various settings in nature – on the coast or in the forest. We brought people together to share skills with each other about beekeeping, beach fishing, weaving, painting, breadmaking, jewellery making and more. It was an abundant system of knowledge transfer and when a class went really well, in an almost supernatural way, we would say it was a magic moment workshop. This became our shorthand for when people left feeling happier than when they arrived. New connections were formed and new skills were passed on – sparks of fun and resourcefulness and inspiration.

From these grassroots days, we noticed something amazing. People told us our classes helped them feel good: less worried, more open, less depressed, more curious. They showed up to learn how to keep bees and how to sew, then told us that being deeply immersed in the process of 'making' gave them respite from tricky states such as stress, anxiety, depression and overwhelm.

When local GPs and psychologists reached out to let us know that they were referring their clients to our classes, it confirmed that we had developed a form of creative prescription, where the very act of making was having a profound and medicinal effect.

Making the shift

In 2019 we shifted our focus, launching a pilot creative prescription group program for people who were no longer able to work due to psychological injuries they experienced at work. ReMind was the first program of its kind. It took participants through an exploration of a range of creative practices such as writing, music, cooking and drawing, while also teaching them how to get to know their own nervous systems and understand what they needed to meet their own social and emotional needs.

Participants told us this was making a real difference, after a long time when nothing else had. We met each week in our local art gallery, and instead of sharing stories about their personal trauma, asked them to play the song they just wrote or share a drawing they just created. Some of those people still meet for coffee to this day.

Let's add a global pandemic!

From 2020 to 2022 – the most intense years of the pandemic – our local face-to-face work had to hit pause. We transitioned our ReMind program online, and an unexpected silver lining was that we could now work with people across the country. Initially designed for people on workers compensation, the program eventually became open to any community members looking to manage their mental health. We unexpectedly found ourselves working with many first responders, mostly police officers navigating workplace-induced trauma.

Each week we would dial in to Zoom and be connected in that box of grids. Jim dialled in from the psychiatric ward; Sam was on leave from working at a maximum-security prison; Graham had post-traumatic stress disorder (PTSD) after witnessing a homicide with no support and was being medically retired from the police force; and Joni, a solicitor, suffered vicarious trauma from working on multiple sexual abuse cases. No-one talked about depression or trauma or anxiety, though, as we were on Zoom together to play the ukulele!

Fingers explored frets and pressed down clunkily to make half-chords, songs were scratched out on paper and an attempt at strumming in unison was made, swiftly cascading into laughter. Someone cried, as did another, then they laughed. Musician Elana Stone was there through it all, humbly encouraging us and tending to our clumsy efforts. Music was managing our emotions and the medicinal impact of this Zoom call was astounding.

In our Zoom workshops, there was almost always an animal or three in the grid. Dogs sat on laps, cat tails swished across the screen, paws clicked on keyboards. Once a parrot flew across the room. There have been guinea pigs, a lizard, a snake, rabbits, fish, chickens and even a large horse in a paddock. Creatures all holding space for their person – for the whole group – for us! For one whole hour, creativity was the prescription... and it worked.

At the end of every eight-week workshop, we witnessed participants metamorphose; for many it was a transformational experience, helping them manage their symptoms, heal and recover. It's what our program evaluations told us with crystal clarity, too. So we've written this book to give you, the reader, an opportunity to understand the intention and purpose of creative first aid, and then explore a library of prescriptions that can offer you the same possibility of transformation.

Creative prescribing in action

Today, our work at MakeShift brings together two key elements. Firstly, we present tools and content that make the case for play as an act of restoration, sharing how our nervous system works, what it needs, and how we can pay attention to that for our own psychological benefit. We share the belief that self-care is a radical act of non-negotiable repair in a culture that prioritises work, and that being creative is required to step outside of 'the way things are'.

Secondly, we invite trusted, contagiously effervescent creatives who inspire others to playfully try out their artistic form in a way that's about the practice being good for you, not requiring you to be brilliant at it. This hands-on creativity brings the theoretical idea of creativity as medicine to life, allowing people to actually feel the impact that being creative has on their body and nervous system, leaving an imprint that lasts beyond the workshop experience.

We've adapted the content and tools of our programs and delivered them in a multitude of ways. We've run a weekly arts-on-prescription program for young people in juvenile justice. We've visited communities reeling from bushfires and floods and put balls of clay – literally soil and ash – into the hands of traumatised residents, listening as they shared their stories while shaping talismans for a community sculpture. We've gone into post-Covid lockdown workplaces, bringing a hundred managers together to draw one another, the laughter so loud no-one could hear themselves think.

We share the belief that self-care is a radical act of non-negotiable repair in a culture that prioritises work.

It's pretty tricky to measure the KPIs of joy in an evaluation report. It's hard to capture the moment when someone's nervous system remembers the feeling of connection and creativity. But this happens every day in our work.

Without applying the practice of creativity to our work, there's no way we would have lasted ten years in business together or achieved all that we have. Our offices are located in an old industrial warehouse that used to house bikie gangs, but is now home to a bunch of artists and creatives. All our work is born here, designed and drafted on laptops and butcher's paper; more often than not, it happens while we're lying on the floor.

For us, creativity has played the role of a friendly companion, one that challenges and supports us, just like the best kind of friend does. It's been something that has helped us mop up tears, had us in deep-belly hysterics, lifted us from flat and lonely moments, and been a constant ignition for ideas and plans. Running MakeShift is a giant creative process; it has its fair share of challenges, snippets of discomfort and 'grumpy struggles',[1] but they are outweighed by moments of deep joy and elation. All of our meetings begin with a five-minute dose of play – anything from drawing each other without looking at the page to squishing clay in our hands to make a pinch pot. It calms any nerves, brings us all into the present moment and nearly always makes us laugh. Creativity is a great prelude to talking about budgets and marketing, and lodging forms with the Department of Fair Trading.

Growing from a grassroots partnership doing small and local work to delivering national programs to thousands of people from all walks of life has been a heck of a ride. Together with our personal experience, we bring a combined four decades of knowledge about cultural and community development, social work, adult education, sustainability activism, arts programming, group facilitation and personal lived experience to each and every one of our programs. We've learnt a lot and we want to share some of that with you here. Our approach and message are always the same: we are all humans, and all humans need to play.

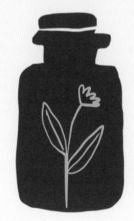

The path that led us here

Caitlin's story

In 2017, Lizzie and I had been running our grassroots community organisation for almost five years. It was fun, creative and so far from the crisis support roles of previous years. I felt the pull to also find some other work to sharpen up my social work and training facilitation skills.

So on a sunny Thursday in November I found myself in a small, windowless, barred room of a correctional facility observing a training session for nurses on vicarious trauma management. I would soon be delivering this training myself many times over for Full Stop Australia.[2] Having lived through fairly seismic vicarious trauma[3] as a young social worker working in sexual assault support services, I spent the day nodding in furious agreement and marvelling at the strategies laid out in the training. They lined up so neatly with the work I'd been doing with Lizzie – nervous system support through self-care is key!

When the nurses were asked to share what they do for self-care, they couldn't think of anything. 'Pick up a six pack on the way home,' joked one. 'Does Netflix count?' chimed in another. They'd just watched a presentation about the role of creative, somatic and relaxation exercises in regulating the nervous system. 'I wouldn't even know where to start with doing something creative,' a third finally said.

This was a lightbulb moment for me. After years of running classes designed to help people explore their creativity, I knew that it quickly brought people to a sense of playfulness and fun. It's healing. It opens up connections. That is, if you know how to flex your creative muscle. 'We need to find a way for people to find this part of themselves, safely, without focusing on being good at it,' I wrote in my notes. 'We need to bring people into a space a bit like kindergarten where there is time to just explore and play and try things and see how you like them. This is a right for everyone, not just those with the time and money.'

This interest in the connection between play, nature and social impact has been a constant thread in my life and work. As a socially anxious, chronically shy kid, I dove deep into consuming music, comedy and musicals. Playing the piano kept my inner life rich and exciting, while slipping under the radar out there in the actual world. Where I grew up in suburban Brisbane (Meanjin), our house backed onto bushland, meaning I spent hours and days in the creek unsupervised, catching tadpoles, riding bikes and picking mulberries.

Inspired by the activism of my mother and aunties – essential for surviving the political climate of Brisbane in the 1980s[4] – I was pulled towards studying social work (though secretly pining for music or art school, and it was no accident that I spent all my spare time hanging around in student theatre, making plays, sets and friends). My first social work job was housing young women who were escaping violence in supported accommodation, and because I was working for a community-run feminist women's service, i.e. a flat structure with no boss, I was given a lot of freedom.

I leaned into my interest in creative practices, and programmed the very same activities I did with my friends, from candle-making classes to T-shirt printing. My clients were all reeling from years of trauma, and these afternoons of creating together brought down the guarded walls for these young women, helping them forge new friendships and feel 'normal' for a few hours.

I also took groups on outdoor education camps. Sometimes we'd go kayaking. Other times we'd traverse ropes courses, where the women would be counted on by their peers to literally hold them up safely through the belay rope. After needing help from others for so long, this single act sometimes changed the way these women saw themselves from that point onwards.

My favourite part of these weekends was the Magic Dinner, where each person was invited to dress up. A taffeta dress, a bow tie and braces, a giant fascinator – silly and ridiculous on purpose. We would guide them into the dining hall that had been decked out with fabric and fairy lights, the long table decorated with tealight candles and vases filled with flowers. The delight in their eyes and on their faces? Magic.

Through this experience, I saw, firsthand, people who went home different from how they arrived. Lighter. Hopeful. Something big had shifted. There was bounce, awe, wonder and connection. I will never forget when 17-year-old Rose, emerging from years of living with an abusive father, looked at me with wide eyes across this Magic Dinner table and said, 'No-one has ever gone to this much effort for me before.'

Rose was used to filling out emergency relief forms and housing applications. She expected to see doctors and counsellors and case workers. Her weeks lurched from crisis to drudgery, waiting for services and trying to rebuild her life. What was wholly unfamiliar to Rose was having a moment of fun, of being treated as someone with something to offer rather than a problem to be solved. Playfulness offered her a little moment outside of her life. Rose held herself differently after that dinner and, in fact, in the weeks and months afterwards. She had experienced a moment of being someone other than a survivor of violence. She literally tried on a different outfit and felt the possibilities for her future unfurl before her. It wasn't everything, but it was definitely something. And it showed me that intentional efforts to bring play, awe, silliness and dressing up into the lives of people as they navigate serious hardship is something to take seriously.

Through my work I've met young folks overcoming heroin addiction, women fleeing violence, families navigating poverty, newly arrived refugees, and people living with complex trauma. I've also encountered many professionals reeling from the cumulative distress that comes from working for overstretched and under-resourced systems.

Artistry is found on stages, in galleries, museums, festival tents. Creativity? It's absolutely everywhere. I often recall a sweet, down-on-his-luck young client I had while I was working at a court-ordered methadone program in Edinburgh, Scotland. Rob couldn't read (and I would coach him in the corridor about what his program report said before we headed into court each month), but wow, could he make me laugh. In his thick Scots brogue and fast banter, he had a running commentary on the obscenely frilly collars and curled wigs of the judges. It would be my turn to stand up in my op-shop 'court jacket' and advocate on his behalf and I'd be wiping away tears of laughter.

Rob knew he was funny, and it was his personal creative expression. Living in the city that's home to the largest annual comedy festival in the world, this sad irony was not lost on him. 'It's okay, hen, I save my best jokes for my social workers, not some crummy crowd of tourists and festival wankers.' I told him he could one day try doing stand-up. 'Ah, that's not for my kind, darling. Leave that to the fancy folks.' Maybe in an alternative universe, he would have been headlining at the Spiegeltent. This brought home to me the stark sense that many people have creative inclinations but can be 'locked out' because of their social status or circumstances.

These experiences have firmly instilled in me the belief that humans are extraordinary and their own creativity can always be found, if you go looking.

They can be softened by kindness and seek out laughter, often, and in the face of tremendous challenges they continue to be curious, make much of very little resources, create connections, and transform.

I also know that when I've had to weather storms in my own life – from up-and-down anxiety, vicarious trauma in my early twenties and the hormonal horror-show that is premenstrual dysphoric disorder (PMDD), to the complex grief that planted itself deeply following the loss of my mother, almost right at the same time that I became one – creativity is the tool I've turned to again and again. Music, nature and drawing remain my trusty, evergreen friends.

I don't fit the stereotype of someone in the helping profession who talks about wellbeing. I'm not softly spoken and neatly held together. I'm messy, and often a mess. My days are soundtracked by constant music – loud and visceral – especially when I'm busy and frayed from the juggle of life. I like fast, slapdash drawing with charcoal and watercolours, and hectic freestyle cooking using every single saucepan and requiring one hell of a clean-up job. My overly busy brain craves big, bold sensory experiences like what I call 'turbo gardening' – pulling out resistant weeds and hauling bags of mulch. All of these things reduce the regular experience of heightened, activated fight-or-flight feelings that my own nervous system is quick to zip to in the face of losing control, stress or Big Life Stuff. I only know this because I've learnt to apply these activities in the moments when they count. Over time, I have learnt what works for my own personal flavour of weirdness.

That is why I share this, by the way: because I believe that every one of us has our own unique set of things that can calm our nervous system. You don't need to 'perform' creativity, you just need to be yourself. You do you, as they say.

That's what is being required of me each and every day now, as I write this book, while navigating the tricky roads of mysterious, relentless chronic joint pain, and also being thrust into what is known as the 'sandwich generation' – parenting two children as well as micro-managing the path of full-time nursing care for a beloved parent. It can bring me into a 'sorry for myself' default setting, especially as the only sandwiches I can actually eat right now involve sponge-like, gluten-free, non-inflammatory bread.

I do know with certainty that you never ever regret a swim, and that plunging into a body of water is the best cure for a hangover, for life grumps and actually many other ailments, too.

Lizzie's story

I was born on Ngunnawal Country in Canberra. Upon arriving in this world, I had a sliding door moment with Caitlin – we were both born in the same hospital, six months apart, with the same obstetrician present, Dr Cutter (what a name!) – but we wouldn't meet for another 30 years.

When I was five, I came home from kindergarten and declared that I had learnt a new word. 'Tintinnabulation,' I told my mother. 'Tintin what?' she asked. 'It means the ringing of bells,' I told her. 'I would very please like to hear the ringing of bells. Where do I find tintinnabulation?' It wasn't the actual sound of bells ringing that I wanted to hear over and over again, it was the feeling that came with learning a word such as tintinnabulation, a word so fine that its onomatopoeic nature matches its musical meaning and conjures up all sorts of twinkly feelings. It was this twinkly feeling that I sought.

Later, in my teens, I learnt that life can be really crap and deeply beautiful all at once. The practice of hunting down a twinkly feeling (what I now think of as a glimmer) has been a throughline in my life and work. You'll read more about the wonder of glimmers in Chapter 3.

I stand in the middle years of life these days, the so-called sandwich years, which makes me think of a sausage sizzle… but as a vegetarian, I'm opting for a tofu burger. I'm a queer white woman with a rainbow family – two mums, two boys, one spaniel.

Before my boys came along, I had a miscarriage. I lost my first little baby in a pool of blood and I ended up in Emergency. I cried as much as I bled, and became anaemic for some time after. Days after I had returned home from hospital, my belly hollow and heart heavy, Caitlin turned up with a plant and a piece of lino. She held space for my discomfort through craft. We didn't talk about the baby I was no longer growing, but she carved a bird and I carved a whale and we printed it DIY-style on the kitchen table. Ink got everywhere, but making these lino prints helped me begin to process my pain and dilute the despair I was feeling at the time. Joy crept in as medicine and a tiny glimmer of it was all I needed to keep going (as well as some iron tablets). A small part of MakeShift was born that day. Over time these tiny pieces of the MakeShift jigsaw puzzle came together to form what it is today.

In early childhood I moved from Canberra to Sydney. Then, soon after I'd turned 13, due to many complex circumstances, my family moved to Hong Kong and it was a tricky time. I spent three years missing home, my older siblings and my friends. I'd dart through busy streets feeling lost. But Hong Kong was also the place where I remember experiencing creativity as a form of medicine for the very first time.

One day I met my friend Mike for lunch in a small restaurant down a laneway full of cafes and shops that sold produce by the bucketful. Baskets of eggs, live turtles floating in barrels, pigs' trotters by the bunch – it was quite thrilling in its unfamiliarity. Mike had brought with him his camera, an SLR with a new roll of film (back in the days when every photo counted!). He handed me his camera and told me to keep it for the afternoon. 'Shoot some photos,' he told me. 'Use the whole roll if you like. We can develop them tomorrow.'

I felt like I'd been passed a piece of treasure and a pair of wings. I spent the whole afternoon on the hectic and bedazzling streets of Hong Kong chasing light and shadows. My eyes followed strings of red hanging lanterns and zoomed in on woven baskets stuffed full of wildflowers. I was beguiled by stray dogs and rows of dried flattened ducks hanging from shop windows. I snapped a whole roll of film in two hours and felt wild and free for the first time in many months. I was utterly and happily lost to the process of taking photos.

This remedy of photography came home with me to Australia, where I completed my final years of schooling. On weekends I took myself to the early morning fish markets, photographing the bustle of giant crates of fish arriving off boats. There were rows of prawns and fish on ice, the sunrise glistened and fishmongers carried armfuls of sea-life to vendors. It was fast-paced, salty, fishy and exciting. I went there to find the feeling of freedom that I'd tasted on the busy streets of Hong Kong. Creativity, like an anchor, was becoming something I could rely on to keep me grounded and interested in life, and dilute anxiety.

After leaving school, I studied English literature and also found my way into a darkroom, my own mind blown developing negatives for the first time. University gave me an enormous stack of black-and-white photos, the salve of poetry, a deep dive into student activism and an arts degree.

From my days in the darkroom full of passion to fight for the planet, I joined and worked for Greenpeace. Learning about international environmental campaigns opened my eyes to the wider world, and from there I found my way to Ladakh, a high-altitude village nestled on the Tibetan plateau. I lived and worked in this remote, mountainous land and it became a transformational experience, glimpsing a life of deep contentment through the lens of a truly sustainable community.

Ladakh smells of donkey dung, goats' milk, rancid butter, animal wool, freshly plucked apricots and glacial meltwater. It sounds like swishing barley grass, bellowing cows, fluttering prayer flags, monastic bells and the stillness of a trillion stars. Daily living is an interplay of creativity, spirituality and inter-generational community connection. Children are raised by friends and extended-family members; education is place-based, and ritual and ceremony are woven into almost everything. It is a truly localised way of life and there is literally no waste. This ancient indigenous culture taught me the lesson of connection. I had travelled halfway across the world, couldn't speak the language, but had never felt so at home and so connected. I would stay up late into the night churning butter by hand; by day I would gather wild apricots. I was immersed in a truly sustainable way of life, so uniquely attuned to the environment and people. It changed me. Ladakh taught me, from the inside out, that creativity is inherent to being human and that spirituality can happen alongside a pile of cow dung! If I were to map my path to MakeShift, Ladakh and all that I learnt there would be one of the most significant plot points.

I returned to Australia committed to living and working with the remnants of what Ladakh had taught me. However, life back home was a far cry from the lowly call of a hybrid yak and flapping prayer flags, and instead saw me train as a certified yoga teacher. I taught yoga to pregnant women and corporates, eventually running private classes at an exclusive boutique retreat. Later I went on to help establish a sustainable living centre, the first of its kind in Australia. The power of community always stayed with me.

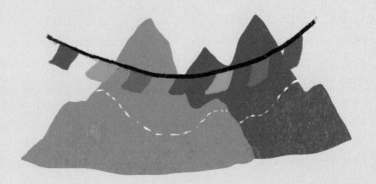

My role at the centre was to bring people together to learn about sustainability – growing veggies, making cheese, building worm farms and compost systems. I coordinated volunteers and teachers, and connected people in community gardens and backyards. I also spent time working in regional towns advocating and campaigning for backyard bird diversity and habitat. I worked with a lot of multicultural communities in this space and we used creativity to connect. Sharing and cooking recipes together, swapping seeds or excess produce, and sewing harvest bags made from scrap fabrics – the innate nature of creativity made it possible to connect no matter what language barriers were in place.

Collating what I have learnt working in Himalayan barley fields, backyards, community gardens, a food co-op, yoga studios and various non-profit organisations, and applying it, alongside Caitlin to create MakeShift, has been a creative practice in itself – weaving the threads of community, connection and creativity into the heartbeat of the organisation. I have co-designed our programs with a personal understanding of trauma, and the MakeShift framework stems from almost three decades of working in social change and community development. My interest has always been in humans and the environment, about the community we live in and the community around us.

For me, this book is a testament to creativity as a reliable guide for life.

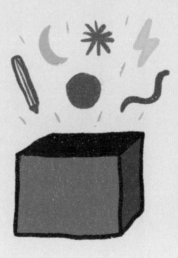

Creativity is within all of us

Creativity as a form of medicine is a movement happening in tiny ways all over the world, gaining momentum in clinic rooms, hospitals and community centres. In Scotland, GPs are starting to prescribe joining a choir to patients who are isolated and depressed. A public hospital in Taipei has established an art gallery program for dementia patients.[5] The New York Society for Ethical Culture now hosts a virtual, global and free storytelling circle, which gathers people around the globe to escape into worlds with fairies, monsters and far-off places, and has been shown to reduce anxiety and isolation for its attendees.[6] Creativity as medicine is not a new idea. First Nations people here in Australia have used dance for more than sixty thousand years as a way to share cultural knowledge and promote health and wellbeing.[7]

It's worth noting that this approach is distinctly different to art therapy. Creative first aid is about the impact that practising creativity for fun has on the rest of our life. Unlike art therapy, it's not using artistic activities to work through therapeutic goals. We'll explore this in more detail in Chapter 2.

One of the biggest gaps in our social literacy about mental health is knowing how our nervous system operates. The act of 'regulating' or adjusting our automated responses to stress is actually the key to wellbeing.[8] Having a regulated nervous system puts us in a space to make good, logical decisions about what else we need, such as eating well, going to therapy or taking some time off work. It's a crucial step in any therapeutic recovery journey for psychological healing. We'll dive into this in Chapter 4.

There has never been a more pressing time to be discussing our mental health and what we can do to improve it. The climate crisis, the Covid-19 pandemic and subsequent lockdowns, hugely divisive political climates, the addictive nature of social media, the cost-of-living crisis – it's quite a time we are living in. A time that means it can be very hard to maintain and protect our mental wellbeing. And on top of everything else, our mental health system is beyond capacity and people are waiting longer than ever to get the support they need. And then, of course, there are the absolutely overworked practitioners who are feeling an enormous strain. This situation is not unique to us here in Australia, it's happening all around the world.

Why practise creativity?

When practised as a tool for wellbeing, we see creativity as a powerful, affordable and accessible way to cultivate care for ourselves, for each other, and for the planet we inhabit. There are six important elements that make this possible:

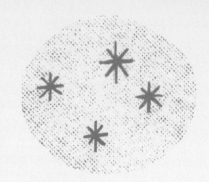

1

Any practice or pastime that combines sensory input and the potential for a state of flow, or play, and that connects with an expression of ourselves that we can't necessarily find words for, immediately **helps regulate our nervous system**. We'll go into more detail about this in Chapter 4.

2

Creativity gives us space to **find meaning beyond our inner world**. It can help cultivate a deep connection to nature and the wonder of the world. It's a portal for the inexpressible, and is something human beings have been exploring for thousands of years.

3

Engaging in a creative activity provides space to practise things like **risk-taking, failure and bravery**. It can build the confidence to be able to do these things in our everyday life and relationships.

4

Turning something we love into a habit also fills the important role of **regularly reconnecting us to glimmers of joy, awe and wonder**. This can offer a welcome perspective when the world feels big and overwhelming.

5

Having a creative practice and an open mindset also helps prime us to be able to **connect to others with empathy** and grounded compassion, enhancing the possibility for greater community care and support.

6

When combined, these elements give us greater capacity to **tune in to our own internal wisdom** and be connected with our body, not just our mind.

The wonderful thing about practising creativity is that it doesn't involve waiting lists or filling out forms. It doesn't even need to cost you any money. You can do it when and where you want, and it can take minutes, not hours. Finding a creative habit, whether it's drawing a self-portrait or making biscuits, that fills you up with warm fuzzies might not be the only answer to improving mental health, but in our experience – and we've had plenty of it – it can change your life!

We hope that by sharing our stories, our methodology and how we use creativity as a kind of medicinal remedy, we can reveal the knowledge behind the academic studies and jargony health service plans. We want to place this knowledge in your hands, just like a ball of clay, so you can have a play, explore and ultimately figure out how this might work for you.

Play is a serious business

Practising creative first aid pulls us into a state of free play, or flow – a human experience that is, as it turns out, essential. Dr Stuart Brown, from the US National Institute for Play, has stated that play is the polar opposite of depression, not work as we might expect.[9] Finding something you love to do – for fun, for connection, for expression – is vital for us humans, and always has been. It doesn't seem to necessarily matter what it is – whatever floats your particular, specific boat. Our work at MakeShift has brought us into contact with people who found their depression and anxiety lessened when they joined a choir, or discovered anime, or got really into Brazilian jiu-jitsu wrestling. There is no end to the list of ways you can be creative.

Creative First Aid is all about the benefits of actively welcoming moments that spark awe and joy in our lives, as an antidote to those sticky moments of despair, loneliness, overwhelm and fear. When we turn those moments into habits, we see that this creates small glimmers of joy that can cascade, grow and enlarge those sparks of awe into a practice we can rely on, each and every day.

This book is for everyone

This book is for anyone who has found themselves wrestling with anxiety and fear, grief and loss, depression and despair, terror and trauma, even the small seeds of these things. That's most of us at some point, right? It's for anyone seeking ways to deal with their life in ways that don't numb their experiences of the good moments.

If you find yourself languishing on a waiting list for support, or you have multiple caring roles and never enough time to care for yourself, or if you work in the health sector, then this book is for you. It's for anyone who has been told they need to 'practise self-care' but with no clear direction on how to do that, and where to find the time! We've written this book for anyone who loves to play and interact with art, but also for those who feel far from creative. In fact, if you feel that way, this book is mostly for you. We know there are lots of you out there. It's never too late to find your own creativity.

A bird's-eye view

We've written this book to give you the theory of creative first aid, as well as tools for practising it yourself. Chapters 1 to 4 make the case for why creativity is a non-negotiable part of being human. Just as we can't rearrange the limbs on our body, we can't take creative design out of us. It's a part of us. We show you the proof that creative practices stand up alongside other mainstream forms of treatment for a range of challenging experiences. We bring together history, stories from our work, research and scientific evidence, and a set of key principles for practising medicinal creativity that add up to help build the momentum to say: 'Yes, I want to have a go!'

In Chapter 1, we introduce definitions of creativity, as well as a process for how to transform it into creative first aid. This process is a creative practice too, and asks us to shift out of our comfort zone to be able to try new things. But it's good news: we get to shift into the zone of play!

In Chapter 2, we discuss the ways our society currently thinks about and treats common psychological experiences such as anxiety, depression, burnout and trauma. Using a vast body of global evidence, we make the case that creative practice, when applied in the right circumstances, can be a universally available, reliable, free resource. We hope to validate how valuable our own creativity can be, and how harnessing it fits into a broader spectrum of health interventions.

Chapter 3 explores three crucial features of the world around us that work in symbiosis with our own creativity and also wellbeing: joy, nature and community. We explore how the human race has actually used creativity, imagination, storytelling and deep connection to the earth to improve wellbeing for thousands of years. It's only quite recently that we have forgotten these truths and now have to actively seek them out.

In Chapter 4, we take you on a journey through your nervous system, sharing ways to get to know just how it responds to stress, fear, grief and loss, and then we offer some tools to help you manage this.

Chapter 5 includes 50 creative prescriptions that you can try out, experiment with and reflect on. These are tried-and-tested practices that range from quick and urgent micro relief prescriptions, to some deeper recharge and restorative habits. Many of them have been gifted to us by extraordinary artists, makers, naturalists, healers, thinkers and practitioners.

Throughout this book you will also find field notes from people we have worked with at MakeShift whose lives have been changed by creativity. They serve as tales from the front line, where creativity has been prescribed as medicinal first aid for people with depression, anxiety, stress, overwhelm, mental health challenges and PTSD. Many of these people had never picked up a paintbrush, let alone an instrument or writing journal, in their adult lives.

We hope this book gives you a roadmap for how to look after yourself on tough days, amazing days and all the other days in between. It's not a magic fix that will solve a complex diagnosis. It doesn't mean that you won't experience moments of feeling overwhelmed or anxious or depressed ever again. We hope that reading this book and trying some of the prescriptions gives you the space to get your hands dirty, make room for restoration and rest, untangle your nerves, find sparks of wonder, and light up your own creativity. We hope it gives you the knowledge and tools to help keep yourself mentally steady. Being in balance with your nervous system has been described as being at 'home'. We hope this helps open up a doorway to being seen, and finding your way home.

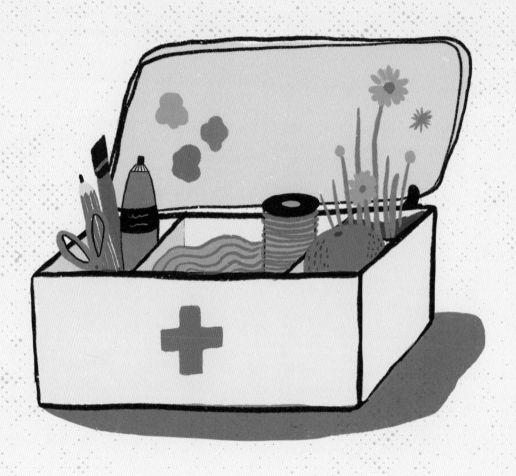

CHAPTER 1

———

Creative First Aid: Creativity is good for us, and we all have it

We have both witnessed hundreds of people experience a noticeable shift in their mental state by interacting with their own inherent creativity. This reminds us of the Japanese word *komorebi*, which describes the awe and wonder of sunlight dappling through leaves, casting dancing shadows and bringing flickers of light to a forest floor. Using art, nature, writing and drawing as a way to navigate the filigree of the nervous system is an approach to life that we have named 'creative first aid'. It is a sort of resuscitation for our creative selves, as a means of care and connection.

Creativity mostly isn't accidental. As a practice, it requires some thought and intention, and transforming acts of creativity into creative first aid for the purpose of connecting us to a moment of pleasure, calming our nervous system and promoting mindfulness requires a plan – a blueprint of core elements. The elements of creative first aid are also innate human practices: safekeeping, playfulness, inch-by-inch thinking, curiosity and self-compassion. Think of them as friends, your own personal cheer squad who've got your back.

In this chapter we get to know these five foundational elements and show you how to work with them to make your relationship with creativity, in whatever way you choose to practise it, one that influences your physical and psychological state for the better. Creativity has the potential to lessen tricky experiences like anxiety, depression, burnout and grief. By drawing upon this innate part of us to play and connect, we can rewire our nervous system in incredibly powerful ways. Using these five elements, alongside a repeated creative practice – even just ten minutes of drawing or having a dance-off in the kitchen – can bring us into a state of mind that helps us feel grounded and able to make good, clear decisions for our health, wellbeing and life.

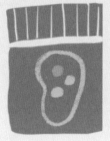

What the heck is creativity?

If what comes to mind when you think of creativity is paints and brushes, or musical instruments, or a craft cupboard, we understand. This is what the concept of creativity has been tied up with for a long time. It's a bit like thinking that physical movement is only about playing football or running a marathon, and that a walk around the block doesn't count as exercise. Limiting the definition of creativity means that many people truly believe they aren't creative. And so if this is you, then it's you we are speaking to, heart to heart. Because you are creative. We all are.

Some might say that creativity is the ability to make art, whether you can write a song or paint a picture. It's the seemingly effortless ease with which you can put pen to paper, sing into a microphone or dance on a stage. People who do those things are definitely creative in ways that define them as artists to be marvelled at. Perhaps their creative expression is even their livelihood. This is one way we witness creativity.

Others might say that creativity is a state of mind that is only for the realm of artists, that it requires the luxury of space and time and inspiration. Perhaps even that creative ideas arrive in one's mind fully formed and it's just a matter of getting them down onto the page, into the aural landscape, into the world. It is an experience reserved for the talented few.

And yet, so many creative acts are performed under devastatingly oppressive circumstances by everyday people. Take, for example, Scottish mountaineer W.H. Murray, who spent three years as a prisoner in World War II. He wrote his book *Mountaineering in Scotland*[1] on scraps of toilet paper, a close-to-finished draft discovered and destroyed by the Gestapo. Or Mostafa Azimitabar, an Iranian refugee who was locked in an Australian Detention Centre when he painted a huge self-portrait with a toothbrush and coffee grounds.[2] The artwork was eventually selected as a finalist for the esteemed Archibald Portrait Prize.

Regardless of circumstance, acts of creativity prevail. Sometimes they are not just acts of creativity but of survival. The ability to be creative is the very thing that cannot be taken away from us humans. We can be imprisoned, removed from our country and family or tortured, but the urge to express ourselves and make things always wins out. It is an essential part of surviving these very experiences.

Our friend, the artist Jack Manning Bancroft, founder of AIME (Australian Indigenous Mentoring Experience) and author of *Hoodie Economics*,[3] articulated this beautifully as we kicked a soccer ball around in his art studio last November: 'The freedom to think anything we want, it's the one thing that the most oppressive regimes in the world have tried to take away, and always fail. [Creativity] is how people can move through these experiences, and it might be all they ever have. Some people will work in terrible jobs and conditions all their life, but they still have this freedom to think, dream, to invent in their minds, to choose.'

Interestingly, the more we try to capture this elusive, mysterious creature, creativity, just like a brilliant, inky octopus, changes form and becomes rigid when under the spotlight. To become its true, fully realised form and character, creativity needs the hands holding it down to just relax and stop insisting on some perfect set of characteristics before it slips away, into the sea.

In the context of our work (and this book), creativity is any act that makes something that wasn't there before – a recipe, a herb garden, a walk around the neighbourhood, a cat meme, a dance move at the traffic lights, a haiku, a moment of movement, a new idea, a mindset. Creativity comes in as many forms as there are people, which is a wonderful thing to behold. It also helps us make connections that weren't there before, linking together ideas, images and concepts.

If we are all creative, why can creativity be so hard?

There is no quality that people are generally quicker to announce their apparent failure at than creativity. It's a curious thing. Despite this innate quality appearing so early in our infancy, we quickly get the message that unless we show exceedingly unusual promise, the correct behaviour is to declare, 'I don't have a creative bone in my body!'

The traditional forms of 'creativity' – painting, writing, making, drawing, acting, storytelling, dancing, playing, singing, etc. – can often have some high fences around them in our weird world. Fences that are designed to exclude. It means that some people who were told they weren't good at singing when they were 13 never, ever do it again.

For many, the memories of dipping their toes in the waters of a creative practice like visual arts or music, dance or performance are ones shrouded in red-hot shame. Facing criticism in those formative years when our brain and sense of self were still very much a work in progress can be one of the cruellest experiences in life. This shame can hang around for decades, stopping us from getting up at karaoke, or saying yes to that life drawing class, or joining a choir. It is a story we have heard thousands of times.

If we line this up alongside sport and exercise, it's easier to see the vast differences in how we are socialised to view creative art forms. Sport is deeply embedded in school and education, with compulsory sports days, events, subjects, carnivals, teams, competitions and awards. We receive these messages so often that people generally don't close the door forever on physical movement. But they do for creativity. Imagine if music, art, dance, writing or comedy were given such focus and resources!

Being 'good' at creativity only matters if it's how we make our living, but otherwise? Can't we release the grip on the need for it to be 'good', whatever that means? In fact, why not embrace the opposite: Shit Craft, Bad Drawings, Terrible Songs, Awful Dancing. Who cares? And the quality is actually a matter of opinion anyway. If it's fun and feels good, why deny ourselves this pleasure?

When we go for a run, we can be untrained, unpractised and unused to it, but we will still get the benefit of the cardio exercise, the peak of endorphins, the rush of adrenaline. It's good for us regardless of whether we're good at it. We can (and should!) think about our creativity this way too. It might be helpful to think of creativity as a muscle, one that needs to be flexed over and over in order to be strengthened.

What is creative first aid?

Creative first aid is an approach to life that uses our innate creativity to protect and support our mental health. Utilising this innate creativity to care for ourselves and others is accessible, sustainable and beneficial.

For example, if you're feeling overcome with anxiety, try filling a blank page with marks – lines, dots, scribbles, whatever you like. This creative act lowers cortisol levels, bringing you back into the present moment and acting as a micro reset. Finding a pause in a flurry of big feelings is where creativity can grow. Creative first aid assists with this expansion, which then expands our capacity to meet life's challenges.

Creative first aid also primes us to be able to connect to others and to form community, a crucial part of what it means to feel safe, grounded and valued. This is the heart of what it means to have wellbeing.

Creative first aid has six main outcomes:

1. It helps to **regulate our nervous system**, bringing our stress responses back into a state of calm.
2. It gives us space to **find meaning beyond our inner world**.
3. It creates a **low-stakes practice ground** for things like accepting failure, managing insecurity and taking risks.
4. It reconnects us to things like **fun, delight, joy, wonder and glimmers** (see page 91).
5. It builds the muscle of joy and delight and **primes us for connecting with other people**, which in turn amplifies our empathy and compassion for others.
6. It combines these elements and helps grow our capacity to **understand the wisdom our body already has** in helping us through life.

These outcomes emerge when we apply creativity using the foundational elements of creative first aid. Sound the trumpets!

The foundational elements of creative first aid

Our methodology of creative first aid comes from a decade of trialling and testing with a broad range of people from all walks of life. We've reviewed them against academic studies and evidence, woven them into our own ethics-approved evaluation and research, and read widely to assess the strength and validity of our approach. We know that these elements also reflect long-used traditional approaches to mental health from many indigenous cultures.[4]

Creative first aid has five foundational elements:

 Safekeeping: minimising any emotional harm when exploring creativity

 Playfulness: no longer focusing on the outcome, instead giving yourself permission to have fun

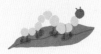 **Inch by inch:** resisting the pull to think in black-and-white terms, instead accepting and celebrating tiny steps in the direction of where you want to go

 Curiosity: cultivating the desire to learn, be inquisitive and look outwards

 Self-compassion: being kind, considerate and generous towards yourself.

We have a plan! The elements of creative first aid in action

Think of these five elements as a treatment protocol. When we get a cold, it's the rest + paracetamol + vitamin C + hearty soup + ginger tea that all band together to aid recovery. When it comes to creative first aid, we don't approach these elements as a list of steps, applying one at a time. Instead, we surround ourselves with these helpful allies and use them to simultaneously support one another and ourselves.

We know this might sound abstract, so let's see how this could work in action.

Overcome with perfectionism to the point where it immobilises you? Does the threat of imperfection trigger a sense of unsafety? Have you ever tried learning a musical instrument? The constant dance with imperfect notes and chords helps us to grow a thicker skin to deal with life's imperfection. It's a great training ground for practising **safekeeping.**

Quick to swing into serious states of fight, flight or freeze at the smallest of things? Try some cold-water swimming. The initial shock to our body and nervous system is only momentary, and quickly brings us back into a regulated state. What's that? A brain-chemically induced high? It's almost impossible not to move about in water, somewhat fish-like, diving and gliding about, so this can be a **playful** space to practise building and adapting to stressful situations.

Feeling frustrated, impatient and wanting things to be different? Try growing a little herb garden. The act of tending to plants helps remind us that things take time, and a little care each and every day can shift things towards the growth we are hoping for, **inch by inch.**

Feeling so anxious that trying new things seems almost too terrifying? **Curiosity** helps us to open doors to things we've never done, assisting us to figure out what we do and don't like. We can try experimenting first with something super simple, such as the creative practice of noticing: *Hmm, look at that cloud... And that bird!*

Doing a lot for other people? For friends, family, pets, neighbours, the planet, but forgetting about yourself? Treat yourself with **self-compassion**, just as you extend compassion to others. Compassion can be cultivated just by giving yourself a moment of time to pause, rest or play.

Applying these elements while at the same time trying out new ways to be creative might feel clunky at first, a bit like learning to drive when you have to talk yourself through all the steps – check the mirrors, step on the clutch, shift the gears, use the indicator. But after a while, that road will have become so familiar in your mind that you'll be able to do these things without thinking. Of course, one of the risks in any kind of prescription can come with its own little wormhole descent into perfectionism, hyper-fixation and overcooking the damn cake. So try to think of these five elements as a bunch of balloons, each one on a string, that you are walking around with. If it's all too much to remember and think about, you can release one, or all of them, just for a time.

By calling forth the five elements at the same time as trying out something creative, we can heal our relationship with our own creativity. Instead of the shame, judgement and a sense of failure that are often the hallmarks of creative expression – whether experienced long ago at school or via a parent – we might connect to a moment of pleasure, calm our nervous system, notice a sense of mindfulness. By gently but intentionally applying these elements, we make these new experiences more possible. We still might sense frustration or discomfort, as is often required when learning and trying new things.

Let's explore each element a little more so that you can start your own journey into creative first aid. Ultimately, discovering how you like to be and feel creative is a unique process. It's a playful voyage that is worth embarking on because it's good for you. So get out those life vests, pals, we're going sailing.

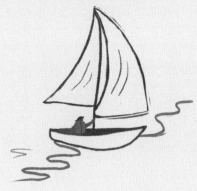

1. Safekeeping

What do you need to feel safe when you're being creative?

Emotional safety is a non-negotiable part of both exploring your own creativity, and growing an understanding of your own nervous system and how it responds to stress, threat and challenges. We will be looking at how this nervous system exploration can happen in the next chapter.

When we feel psychologically unsafe, it changes the way we behave, think and feel, pushing us into survival mode with guarded protections that are great for the short term but can make it harder to feel able to express ourselves freely. We may experience these protections as a feeling of dread in our gut, or as our heart rate increasing, pounding in our chest. Or we might suddenly feel irritation and anger, and our breathing may speed up. When we are forced into a situation that feels very out of our control, or triggers feelings from a past experience that colour and infuse the present, we can lose our sense of emotional safety. For some people, being asked to do 'something creative' can prompt this response, recalling memories of being shamed or humiliated by formative expressions of our own creativity.

We've heard many tales of childhood piano lessons where a wrong chord meant a rap on the knuckles with a feather duster. Or a student's landscape drawing held up and publicly scorned at art school. It's hard to imagine how these learning environments could ever be expected to produce good work.

Here are a few tips to bring forth this practice of safekeeping when you begin a new creative activity:

* Create a space that is private and in your control.
* Make the space feel cosy – maybe you are wrapped in a blanket, listening to music or sitting in the sun, with a cup of tea at the ready.
* Set yourself a time to be creative – 'I will try this [practice] for 20 minutes.'
* Start with some deep, calming breaths.
* Notice any tension, fear or worry and acknowledge it. See if you can let it pass you by.
* Start your creative activity.

Creative first aid offers a space for practising things that can feel unsafe, such as expressing ourselves, or taking a risk, or trying something new. This, in turn, can help us face the outside world. Creativity is also a practice that strengthens the more we do it, and it can help us grow, improve and ultimately enjoy a new part of ourselves.

Practice doesn't make perfect!

The verb *practise* literally means to do something regularly in order to get better at it. We all start out being complete beginners at whatever it is we want to learn, be it a musical instrument, a language or how to make a soufflé. Most things in life require us to do them over and over before we become solid and confident and good at them.

There is also just the most delightful thing about the double meaning in the term 'creative practice'. Taking up a creative habit gives us a training space to practise for difficult situations and experiences that life asks of us – trying new things, living with imperfection, dealing with stress and being uncertain – which in turn *builds safety*.

Safekeeping does not mean guaranteed comfort. Going to therapy is uncomfortable, but so very needed sometimes. Getting to know your creativity can also be uncomfortable. We can work to keep ourselves as safe as possible while learning something challenging. In fact, sometimes we need discomfort in order to learn and grow, to expand and stretch. However, discomfort can be softened if we dial up our sense of playfulness.

Taking up a creative habit gives us a training space to practise for difficult situations and experiences that life asks of us.

2. Playfulness

How can you bring more play into your life?

Research has shown that without play, adults are less curious, less imaginative, and can lose a sense of joyful engagement in daily life.[5] Playfulness is a state that removes expectation and pressure to achieve a certain outcome. It's a quality that's about curiously exploring something for no particular reason at all, and is therefore so essential as we use creativity to offset tricky feelings and experiences.

The founder of America's National Institute of Play, Dr Stuart Brown, noted that studies show 'if they are well fed, safe and rested, most mammals will play spontaneously.'[6] Not too long after we're born, most of us learn to grasp with our hands. We reach for a pen, pencil, texta or crayon with chubby, keen fingers, confident in our clumsiness. Soon after, we figure out that this tool can make a mark. It's exciting! We draw lines, dots – sometimes obsessively – on paper, our bodies, the walls. We draw in the sand, make lines in the steam from the shower; we draw with our food, smashing pumpkin across the table. We are almost primal in our urge to make a mark. It's something that predates verbal language; we are literally hardwired to draw.

So why, then, do we stop? If you watch a child, the pathway from thinking to drawing is seamless, unfiltered, free and playful. Most of all, it happens without that all-too-familiar voice saying, 'You can't draw, you're not an artist.' But something happens in our culture when we become adults. We stop scribbling, singing, moving and creating for the sheer fun of it. We get busy and, often without even realising it, we leave playfulness behind.

That busyness is one of the leading reasons that experts believe we have such soaring rates of mental health challenges – we've created lives with no time and space for play. One of the hallmarks of play is that it lacks purpose, it's just for fun, for no reason. Activities like resting, daydreaming and doodling are often viewed as unproductive, and the pastimes of idle, unserious people. We can't monetise playing, because the possibility of play is immediately removed once there is an outcome or achievement required. The very essence of play is an absence of these conditions.

As we say at MakeShift, play is a serious business. What's serious about it is the primal impulse that it comes from, play being part of our essential biological design, as it is for all mammals.[7] Play is a type of rest state for our brain and nervous system and body. We need it – it's a part of our biology that's as important as nutrition, exercise, safety and sleep,[8] and instead of it being a thing we only do when life is dandy, it's essential that we cultivate it purposefully when times are tricky, too.

The psychological concept of 'flow' or the notion of 'being in the zone' is the essence of what it means to be at play. Coined by Hungarian–American psychologist Mihaly Csikszentmihalyi, 'creative flow' is described as 'a state in which people are so involved in an activity that nothing else seems to matter; the experience is so enjoyable that people will continue to do it even at great cost, for the sheer sake of doing it.'[9] Being in a flow state requires relaxation (don't try too hard to find it!) and a quieting of control, critique and judgement. Feeling safe and curious helps set the stage for this state of play or flow to be possible.

Play also builds muscle memory, enabling us to engage without thinking too much about the process. As poet Jaya Savige notes, 'Climbers, surfers, as well as musicians, rappers and so on must develop technique – or "chops" let's say – while at the same time, they know that being too cognisant of technique can lead to disaster (by interrupting "flow" ...) and so they aspire to a kind of forgetting when it comes time to act ... But this "forgetting" is paradoxical: a kind of forgetting that permits traces of memory.'[10]

The feeling of being stuck or blocked or hitting a wall can be the signal that our internal pendulum has swung away from playfulness. This can be the reminder to return to play.

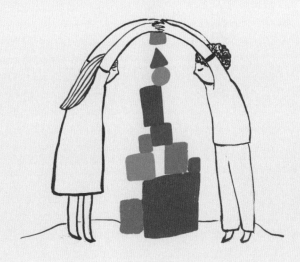

3. Inch by inch

How can you step one inch closer to your own creativity?

Inch-by-inch thinking reminds us that we don't need to set ourselves unachievable goals that we will no doubt fail to meet. It's about replacing binary thinking – well or unwell, on or off, good or bad – and instead viewing our actions, goals and thought patterns on a spectrum. This spectrum is one in which we can celebrate micro steps that inch us towards a place of comfort, safety, kindness and playfulness.

We can be easily wooed by stories of big change, and also feel motivation to make overly ambitious life transformations that often trip us up as we're getting started. Before and after photos. Big reveals. Bold, dramatic change impresses us, especially when it comes to our health and wellbeing. We crave it, while fearing it at the same time. Of course we do: it's exciting, dangerous and energising.

When life feels tough or messy, we can yearn for things to be different. It can be tempting to wish for a fast-forward button to transport us to this future where everything has changed (for the better, naturally!). Even imagining that possibility is creativity in action.

But the truth is, change rarely happens like that. Instead – and this is especially true when it comes to changing our behaviours or thought patterns – this kind of change often requires many, many tiny steps. Eventually, those minutes and hours lead to the change we had longed for. But it is not a 'one and done' process, it takes time.

Inch-by-inch thinking is especially useful during those days and moments when judgement, self-critique and fear are particularly present. What can I do right now that is one inch away from those things? How can I make one step towards self-compassion? Towards a moment of play? Taking things inch by inch enables us to feel as though our goals are within reach. One tiny step is just that. It doesn't demand perfection. A bold giant leap does – we need to execute perfect timing, trajectory, force and inertia to make sure we land in the right place.

David Byrne, lead singer of the band Talking Heads, has spoken in interviews about the concept of 'Little Beginnings'.[11] He explains that his songs don't come to him as fully formed ideas. Instead, he collects little beginnings of songs: a line of lyrics here, a five-note melody there. These little beginnings can then be connected, growing into something bigger and eventually reaching a point where: voilà! David Byrne has just written a new song.

Presumably, there were years when David Byrne took no notice of those little beginnings and they were tossed away. It's through years of practice and making music that he's learnt to trust that sometimes those little things can lead to big, meaningful things, but it means trusting in the small inches we make each and every day.

A common mistake is to focus only on the final product of a creative act. The secret that many artists understand is that it is the process itself that is the gift, and it is made up of a thousand tiny steps. It's the experience of actually making art that motivates them to keep doing it. The final product or work being seen by others of course weaves its way into this process – more often than not, artists don't begin with a complete and finished work fully formed in their mind. This is a deep trusting that comes with the doing of it over and over.

Life does call for big leaps sometimes, but in this process of practising creative first aid, we invite you to start inch by inch. Take solace in the little beginnings. Instead of seeing things as an 'on' and 'off' switch, instead we see them as dials that can be enlarged or reduced. Being mindful of when we start getting caught in binary, black-and-white, all-or-nothing thinking can be the prompt to return to inch-by-inch thinking instead.

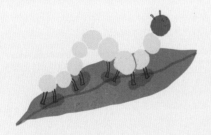

A common mistake is to focus only on the final product of a creative act. But it is the process itself that is the gift, and it is made up of a thousand tiny steps.

4. Curiosity

What would happen if you just gave it a red-hot go?

Curiosity is how play happens. It's how judgement and self-critique can be softened. Curiosity is looking outwards. It is a question, an open-armed wondering. Curiosity is a natural instinct that slowly gets crowded out by perfectionism, trauma and the push to conform. It's the curiosity of a four-year-old that drives parents wild when they are woken at 5 am to be asked if flowers have cousins and if cats would be friends with sloths in the jungle.

There is a rule of thumb in improv theatre called 'Yes, and... ' Basically, this acceptance principle means that the worst possible thing to do on stage in the midst of improvisation is to turn away, say no and shut down an opening. So if your improv partner says, 'Hey, can you hear a braying sound coming from somewhere?', you don't say no. You respond with, 'Oh yes! That's my pet donkey Greg, and he loves having a bath. He's having one right now. Would you like to meet him?' This form of curiosity is generous. It's a hand reaching out, an invitation to see what else might be possible.

As we get older, our curiosity muscle often becomes weaker, but it can be strengthened. Being curious enables us to try out things without deciding first why, how, when and for what purpose: 'I wonder if I like the colour orange'; 'I wonder if wearing swishy pants feels nice.' We probably don't remember asking ourselves these questions when we were ten years old, but we did.

The other gift of curiosity is that it can counteract judgement and a closed mind. Judgement isn't much fun. It is often the force behind our inner critic. Judgement says, 'Don't bother, you won't be any good at this.' A closed mind says, 'Who do you think you are? What a waste of time!' Judgement and shame work together like a gang, out to sabotage really genuine efforts at play and self-compassion.

In fact, shame is the most immobilising of all human emotions. It's what keeps survivors of abuse quiet for decades and keeps people small and obedient. It's the lever that many religions and doctrines have weaponised to keep the faithful in line. Shame is disgust for oneself and, when it comes to creativity, it's perhaps the most powerful voice that haunts those who don't feel creative.

When they try to practise creativity, shame speaks these truly awful words: 'Who do you think you are? Just who do you think you are? Some kind of artist? Pah. But you're terrible.'

By dialling up our curiosity, we automatically dial down the volume of our inner critic. We open the doorway to other possibilities and allow ourselves to get in the zone of play.

Curiosity, when it comes to creative first aid, is about asking 'why', 'how' and 'what if' questions:

✽ Why do I believe I can't draw? What might happen if I just kept going?
✽ How does moving paint around a page feel?
✽ What might happen if I try to write for five minutes?

This permission-giving helps us push through the loud voice of judgement and self-critique, allowing us more time to actually settle in and discover some glimmers and wonder.

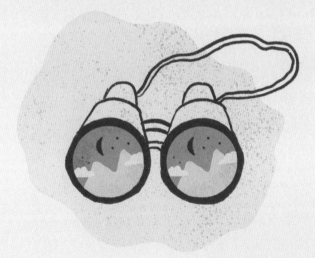

By dialling up our curiosity, we automatically dial down the volume of our inner critic.

5. Self-compassion
What would being kind to yourself feel and look like?

Self-compassion is key in exploring your own creativity. It's the anchor that keeps you from free-falling into judgement and listening to your internal critic, which offers only searing takedowns of any first efforts to make marks, or music, or art. Offering yourself self-compassion is often the first step in changing your life. It's the voice inside you that notices all of your good intentions, knows your heart, and wants you to succeed. It's often a quiet, small voice that can be hard to hear over the roar of others. In fact, many of us are so practised in only hearing this voice's polar opposite – the inner critic – that we don't even recognise what self-compassion sounds like. So here we intend to turn up the volume!

As you begin to explore creativity in a new way, particularly if you are unfamiliar with the practice, it is likely that the voice of your inner critic will be loud. In fact, that loud voice has worked hard to keep you safe from this ordeal for a long time. We all have this voice, which was born of our ancient, primal programming, designed to keep us safe within the tribe, to not stick our head up and be at risk from prey.[12]

One of the first steps in learning to quieten this voice is to recognise it when it shows up. This invitation right here is not a demand to rid yourself of this voice. It will never leave you. Instead, it's an open-armed suggestion to bring to these practices a giant dose of kindness to ourselves. You are trying. You are being brave.

If you tune in to your own voice or sense of the inner critic and really think about how it speaks and what it says, you would probably never dream of speaking this way to someone else. Self-compassion says, 'Hey you, I see you. It's okay. You deserve some peace and calm. You get to play, just like others. Let's give it a go, hey?'

And practising self-compassion isn't just about turning down the volume of that inner critic. It's also about giving ourselves permission to do things imperfectly. And that's important – practising this kind of creativity will be imperfect, always. Consider this your lifetime permission slip!

Practising self-compassion also allows us to get comfortable with the idea that we all contain multiple truths. Humans are complex, flawed and mysterious. We can be unwell and also high-functioning at work. We can be in pain and also look pretty great. We can know that things are bad for us but do them anyway.

Curiosity is a pathway into self-compassion, and vice versa. They are fast friends and they really help each other out. We are not switching off self-critique and switching on self-compassion. That would no doubt just set us up to fail, triggering a visceral rush of judgement and spiralling us away from any kind of creativity at all.

Instead, think about the way we can turn the dial one little notch towards self-compassion, and one little notch away from self-critique. It's an inching that gets easier with practice.

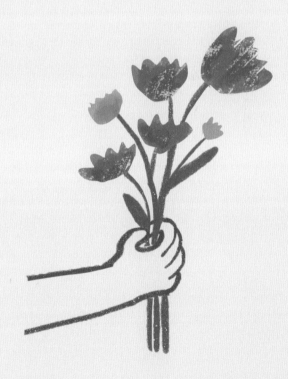

The five foundational elements in practice

To offer a real-life example of the application of these foundational elements, let's meet Nicole.

Nicole was in the Australian Federal Police for more than two decades. Her final years were spent working on serious crimes in the domestic violence high-risk offender team.

'I really liked my work, but the culture of the police was hard. You're meant to be thick-skinned and built to be resilient. Accepting help was not the done thing. So when it got too much for me when I was working with victims, I just didn't know what to do. I was not okay.

'Over my whole 22-year career I got offered counselling once, via email. It said if you want to reach out, then contact this person. It was after I'd been to a pretty bad deceased estate and then later that same day, a homicide. I never did reach out, no-one ever came to talk to me and at that point I was okay. Those cases weren't what I was struggling with, it was years later, after working in the high-risk team with victims, that undid me. It was, like I said, an accumulation.'

We were introduced to Nicole when she joined our ReMind program. She was on a psychological injury claim and unable to work. The story that she shares with us, years later actually, reveals her journey through creativity using the five guiding principles, and the impact this had on her recovery.

'Remember that first Zoom call of the program?' Nicole asks. 'I nearly didn't press "join" that day, I was so scared to log in. I was in a really low place. I'd isolated myself, hadn't left the house. I wouldn't even go outdoors. The ReMind program was my first interaction and it was like my finger slipped on the keyboard and suddenly I'd tumbled into the Zoom room and there you all were, so friendly and welcoming. Gosh, I'm so glad I dialled in that day. I wouldn't be here, where I am right now, if I hadn't done that.'

That nanosecond of **self-compassion** that Nicole gifted herself turned out to be a transformative, life-changing moment for her.

'Since that first Zoom, it's just been **inch by inch** of getting better through art and making. It all really started with the package, I guess. I remember getting a parcel. It was addressed to me, with my name on it, but I couldn't figure out who on earth would send me a ukulele!' she laughs. 'Just being sent those things gave me permission to try things I hadn't done before. It got me **curious** about them.' Nicole is referring to the big, fun box of program materials we shipped out to ReMind participants, that included items such as herb seedlings, a ukulele, paints and writing journals.

It was curiosity that enabled Nicole to try out so many practices in our program. Some things she loved and others not so much, but this was a crucial part of the experience – it gave her a chance to play and feel the sensations of liking and disliking things. This is where curiosity can take us.

'Painting just hooked me right from the start, and took me into another place I didn't know I needed to visit,' says Nicole. 'My nan was a painter. When she passed, my grandfather gave me all of her watercolour paints and brushes. My psychologist challenged me to pick them up and have a go. I wasn't ready then, but later, when I eventually found MakeShift, things clicked. I felt a bit braver and I picked up those paints and had a **play**.

'I felt strange, anxious, scared and shaky, and then when I sat down painting… it felt like magic. I'd be transported into a space of peace and happiness and **safety**. I feel instant calm, relaxed, and everything I'm worried about evaporates and I just think about what I'm doing right then and there. I've never given up on art through all of this PTSD, all the hard days. It's really been my saviour.

'I'm the first police officer in the state, as far as I know, to manage to get recovery funding to engage with and make art for recovery,' Nicole explains. 'You get funding pretty easily if you have a psych injury to go and see an exercise physiologist. I got sent to one for three months, to go to the gym and fitness classes, but it wasn't calming me down or easing my symptoms. Art was, so I never gave up on it.'

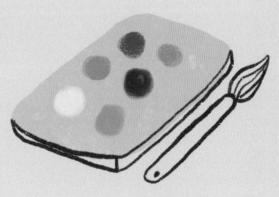

Some notes on trauma

Nature writer and scientist Robert Macfarlane talks about 'trace fossils', a sign left in rock by the impression of life rather than life itself... like a dinosaur footprint. 'A trace fossil is a bracing of space by a vanished body, in which absence serves as sign.'[13]

We can think about trauma in this way, like imprints left behind from life's bruising and devastating moments. These 'traces' in our nervous system can show up, disrupting and wreaking havoc on our life – days, months and even years later – influencing our responses, reactions and relationships, and our sense of self and the world around us. Dr Bessel van der Kolk, a pioneer in trauma research, says that healing from trauma is about learning to live fully in the now.[14]

We know that many people who are navigating daily experiences of anxiety and depression are also survivors of trauma. One of the most important parts of any trauma recovery journey is to learn and understand how to make sense of the way the nervous system responds to trauma triggers. This can be a very effective way of living in the now, and a place where creative first aid can play a role in helping anyone who has experienced trauma.

We are living in a time when new and renewed understandings of the causes, experiences and prevalence of trauma are coming thick and fast. Trauma is a spectrum and can be experienced from one significant event, or the cumulation of circumstances over time.

In all of the work we do at MakeShift, we take what is called a 'trauma-sensitive' approach. This means that we remain sensitive to the fact that a significant number of people have experienced some kind of trauma, and so we offer accommodations for them to be able to participate in creative activities, despite these impacts. A trauma-sensitive approach can look like an intake process where a program participant doesn't have to explain their 'story' multiple times, if ever. Ultimately, this approach respects the agency and wisdom of each and every person in the way they choose to engage with something – a service, a group, an activity, etc. And it actually benefits us all, not just trauma survivors, by offering a range of choices, transparency and sensitivity to the unique preferences of everyone.

One of the key parts of the trauma-literacy movement is being cautious of a requirement to 'talk about our trauma'. When it comes to trauma, discussing it, again and again, isn't often the path to recovery. Trauma is stored in the body and held as a memory. The most effective interventions,[15] as recognised by many trauma clinicians and researchers, are somatic (relating to the body), working to redirect the automatic messages of our nervous system through therapies such as EMDR (eye movement desensitisation and reprocessing) and neurofeedback, and also somatic breathwork, bodywork and sensory experiences.

Creative first aid can work to disrupt and reroute messages to the brain that are activated through an automatic reaction to what can be, at times, almost invisible triggers. Prescribed creative practice can help shape our nervous-system response towards safety. Practising creativity can help us craft new narratives and express ourselves in ways that traditional 'talk therapy' can't.

There is a phenomenon that trauma recovery clinicians call 'post-traumatic growth', which refers to the ways that positive change can occur in the healing of truly traumatic events. One of the key ways this growth can spring forward is in greater creativity, along with closer relationships and increased compassion.[16] The kindness that self-care through creativity can offer survivors of trauma is another key benefit. We often blame ourselves for atrocities inflicted on us that we never deserved, and so building low-stakes creative habits that slowly build self-compassion can help shift this, over time. Accepting the reality that multiple things can be true at once acts like a release valve for perfectionism and instead invites compassion and empathy for ourselves and others. The outcomes of creative first aid that we introduced earlier are all potentially transformative in the journey of healing trauma experiences.

Prescribed creative practice can help shape our nervous-system response towards safety.

Learning to listen to your inner wisdom

One of the things that can make seeking help to deal with trauma incredibly difficult is that many survivors experience a disconnect from their instincts – their inner wisdom, or gut. This is why the foundational elements of creative first aid focus on the idea of safety and safekeeping. For many survivors of trauma, the invitation to 'listen to your body' or 'trust your gut' can be entangled in a knot of confusing urges and messages, especially when the body has learnt to numb sensations and messages as a survival tool, so you don't even know how you feel at all.

When we try to trust our gut but also live in a perpetual state of activated trauma and stress responses, then our gut might tell us lies. It might say, 'Run for your life!' even though there is no need to run. It might say, 'Be small! Be quiet! Stay hidden!' when there is no need to hide. But by simultaneously repairing our nervous system to reset it to our rested, grounded state, and doing something that gets us into that flow state, we inch closer to being able to truly tune in to our gut instinct from a place of deep knowing rather than from fear, threat and stress.

Gently does it

For anyone reading who is recognising themselves here, know that you are worth the time spent on these practices that aid healing. Shifting away from trauma controlling your day-to-day life and reaching recovery is totally possible. If you haven't already, we encourage you to reach out for professional support with a trauma-informed therapist. There are also some reading recommendations on page 257 if you'd like to understand more about trauma and trauma impacts.

This is also a reminder that bringing forth the five foundational elements of creative first aid will take time. Dialling up the kindness to yourself is critical here, as some of the creative prescriptions we share later in this book might feel challenging to begin with. Sometimes this is because play, and free and curious expression, are so unfamiliar to a nervous system that is soothed by tight control and order. The key is to notice those responses, stay curious and go gently.

'Everyone is born creative and every day is an opportunity to perform a new creative act.

When it's hard to paint the clouds we draw the mountains.

Making things makes us feel good.

We learn to do something by doing it.

When we are brave our life expands.

Risk is what transforms us.'

—

**From 'The Imperfect Manifesto'
by Julie Paterson and Manda Kaye**

✳ **Field note** – Crafting as a radical act: Annie's story

In 2021, MakeShift made a podcast called 'In the Making'. It was a compilation of stories from makers and artists who have used creativity as an antidote to challenging times. Annie's story was included in this podcast. One day Lizzie went to visit Annie in her homemade strawbale house, to hear about how she has made an entire life, house and all, from the depths of creativity.

Together, they sat on Annie's daybed covered in crochet blankets, their backs against a wall that had a small crack running down it, which was stuffed with rainbow pompoms. 'Trick of the trade,' said Annie. 'You can stuff anything with a pompom!' With a pot of tea between them and a plate of handmade bickies, Annie told her story while she knitted, with two cats purring on her lap.

'It was 1 am when we woke to a glow in the sky, with alerts and text messages from my family evacuating their homes. Smoke filled the sky, and we watched the glowing horizon as our evacuated family members made their way to the beach. The next day we learnt that as we lay awake with panic rising around us in the hot, glowing windy night, whole towns were burning. My parents-in-law's home burned to the ground.

'Our handmade home was the biggest craft project of my life and also one of the hardest things I'd ever done. My partner and I hand-built a 26-square-metre strawbale tiny home with no running water or electricity, to try out this building caper and get ourselves out of the rental market.

'We were committed to creating a life that was a response to climate catastrophe and the fractured communities of late capitalism. The example my parents had given me – make your own life using your own two hands – seemed both practical and revolutionary, since the hegemonic and heteronormative cookie-cutter lives of consumption and overwork seemed both untenable and profoundly undesirable. We took our lives into our own hands and worked our butts off to forge something different. Something radical and joyful. Something handmade.

'In the midst of all our handmade-life-making, I was, at the age of 35, diagnosed with very aggressive breast cancer, and underwent a bilateral mastectomy as well as several months of chemotherapy. I spent the sunny winter days bundled in blankets, crocheting my heart out, because it was the only thing I could do with my hands.

'Around two years after the cancer situation, we invited 25 friends, family and strangers to come and help us raise the strawbale walls for our home, and then ten months later we slept in our handmade home, our big, collectively handcrafted radical home.

'Living in a handmade home like this is literally living craft every day. Each curve, each piece of timber, each piece of furniture has a story, has been handmade with love. As such, there was never a question for me about whether I'd evacuate or stay and defend in the event of a bushfire. What would our radical handmade life look like if we lost our home, like so many people did during those fires? But the wind changed. And blew the fire in another direction.

'I live in our handmade home, which is my deepest joy and my proudest achievement, and I gather friends and family here, and I wonder that it's been spared. I love her wonky walls and gaps and weird things I botched because I didn't understand. I love that she's still a bit of a work in progress, that I've shown my kids that you can build a life using your hands, and that that life can resist dominant paradigms that dictate that you "can't" or "shouldn't" make things for yourself. That tells you not to try in case the things you make are "bad". That it's better to work in a soulless job so you can pay others to use their hands to make things for you – your clothes, your home, your garden.

'Just over a year before the fire, I was diagnosed with metastatic cancer, spread from my breasts to my liver and bones. My life now is quieter, more gentle, more careful, and more precious. I take medication to control the cancer, I have appointments and blood tests and scans and injections.

'My body is sore, and can't do the things I used to do. My mind is foggy from the meds, and I forget things, including whole conversations. Sometimes it's scary. I sew and knit hectically bright outfits for myself when I have appointments with my oncologist, to brighten the waiting room and provide myself with a symbolic rainbow shield against the bad news that may come. I sew and knit hectically bright outfits for my loved ones because I have a vision of my funeral in which everyone is wearing colourful things that I've made for them. I know that I could never build another home. This is it.

'I believe and have faith that the handmade – which can, in times of disaster, in the face of climate catastrophe and other global traumas, seem so naive, so silly, so small – is still radical.'

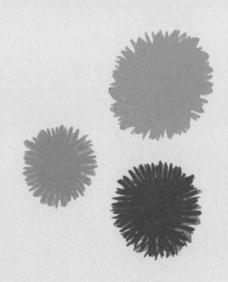

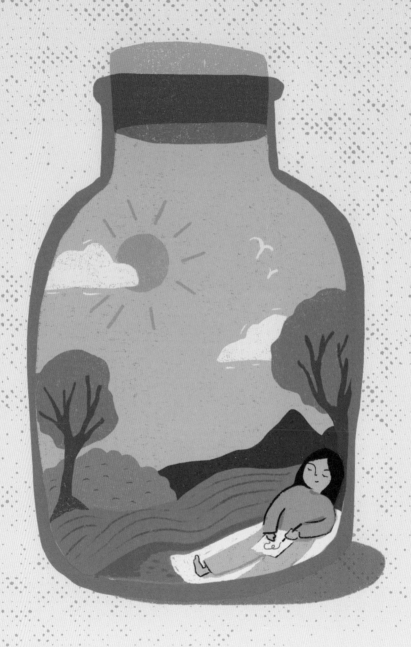

CHAPTER 2

Creativity as Medicine: The science and the evidence

by Caitlin

Throughout this book, we have included many stories about the power creativity can have on improving, supporting and protecting our mental health, but as a reader you might be asking, 'Sure, sure, but where's the science? Show us the proof, Caitlin!' A great question.

In this chapter, we'll look at the proof that at the very least, practising creativity in intentional ways does make a difference to our mood, self-worth, sense of belonging, energy, purpose and social connectedness. We'll explore the compelling results from many small yet valuable research studies dotted around the globe, and we'll spell out how this application of creativity is being delivered in health settings, with incredibly positive outcomes.

Finally, we'll examine the current way that mental health is approached and treated, and highlight the gaps that the medical model of treatment has in truly responding to people's lives and experiences.

Creative first aid works everywhere!

As part of my work facilitating Vicarious Trauma Management training to teams in first-responder workforces for Full Stop Australia, I spent a day with a large team of managers from a federal government agency. One participant approached me at lunch, a sensible, clean-shaven man. He had multiple roles supporting families after child protection reports are made, offering counsel and support to families and survivors. It's a big load to carry. He told me that he has found the key that holds him together, an activity that lessens the impact of hearing traumatic stories over and over: sewing.

He sews to take his mind off things, to keep his hands busy, to focus on stitches one after the other, to meditate rather than allow his mind to dwell on the trauma he experiences at work. Given his workdays can be filled to the brim with loss and absence, it makes sense that creating physical, tangible and useful things feels empowering. From backpack protectors to rain hats, he makes strong, practical items for outdoor use.

It can be easy to dismiss this as a one-off story, but in our experience at MakeShift, this is such a common narrative. Whenever we speak about our work or facilitate a workshop, at least one person sidles up to us afterwards, almost in confession mode, to tell us about their passion for mushroom hunting or opera singing or rug making or how learning the tin whistle 'saved their sanity', or is 'better than therapy'.

Creativity, when practised intentionally, *can* perform the task that actual medicine has been prescribed for. That might sound like a bold statement, but the studies we share in this chapter bear this theory out and show incredibly exciting promise. We've seen this in action and felt it, too. It has even shown up in our evaluation reports, where participants have shared just how much creative first aid improved their mental health, not just during the program, but for months and years afterwards.

Here is where we want to acknowledge multiple truths. Yes, creativity can be medicinal, along with actual pharmaceuticals, too. A bit of guitar strumming might not 'cure' depression, but neither might, as it turns out, antidepressants. Both of those things can help, though, for sure. Creative practice actually plays a vital role in supporting the nervous system to be ready for treatment. It enables us to connect to others, and shifts how we manage our symptoms of mental ill health.

Creative first aid is also incredibly useful for people looking to keep their mental wellbeing steady and healthy. It's for everyone!

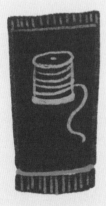

> **'You don't have to be good at art for art to be good for you.'**
>
> **Dr Christina Davies[1]**

Proving it: look, it's complicated

Of course, we must back up all of our claims with science and research. Interventions claiming to help and support people who have experienced trauma or depression need to be applied with care, and tested to ensure that such interventions don't inadvertently cause more harm than good.

While we don't intend to be needlessly controversial, the reality is that given the political landscape of research funding, and the monopoly big pharma has on steering the direction of mental health treatment towards pharmaceutical prescriptions, it can be a little tricky.[2] While there are plenty of studies – hundreds, in fact – that confirm what we have seen over and over in our programs and groups, many of them are small. This is due to the fact that researchers are waiting for support from those with the buckets of money to fund these kinds of studies.

Alison Gopnik, philosopher and psychologist, coined the term 'lantern consciousness' after researching the way babies' brains absorb and process information.[3] While adults tend to focus on one or two things, like a spotlight, babies and small children seem to operate in dramatically different ways. Their minds are able to zoom out, like a drone hovering over a city, noticing the patterns lights make across a vast area, making connections across diverse and different data and inputs in creative and novel ways. This is known as Lantern Consciousness. Light the lanterns!

Building the body of evidence for the role of creative practices in health treatments is a little like searching for small lanterns across the land. Together, when we connect and join them together, they add up to a compelling body of evidence that is, at the very least, worth exploring.

We can start with our own research here at MakeShift. Over a three-year period, 41 people attended our ReMind program. We found that 75 per cent reported significant improvement in their wellbeing, as well as in their own ability to manage their mental health. Participants also showed significant improvement in their depression, with 36 per cent noting a significant reduction in its severity. There was also a marked decrease in anxiety.[4]

Of the participants who began the program stating they had suicidal thoughts most days, by the completion of the program, these participants universally recorded 'no days'. Fifty per cent of participants reported making new social relationships from the program, and 75 per cent felt more hopeful about the future. One group member said 'my confidence has certainly increased in simple tasks, which allows me to help others and feel more valued as a person'.

Is this program a cure-all? No, and we don't believe it should be. In fact, the focus on 'cure' is perhaps unhelpful. Instead, if we apply the concept of inch-by-inch thinking, remembering that multiple things can be true at once, it is often more helpful for people to focus on steps towards recovery. Cure might look like managing an ever-changing mental health status for the duration of one's life, in ways that don't reduce or impair that person's function and participation in their life, rather than the complete erasure of symptoms forever.

While recovery is possible, it most often requires a suite of interventions, tools and strategies. Is having a creative practice the only answer? No, of course not. But it does seem like a possible answer to take seriously. There's enough evidence that tells us this: connecting to something you enjoy, that brings a sense of flow, delight, purpose and play, can lower depression and anxiety. And a clear path to this connection is your own creativity.

Give us numbers!

Okay. Here's some more evidence. Let's go.

Researcher Dr Pippa Burns led a study in 2022 exploring the effects of crochet on wellbeing in more than 8000 survey respondents from around the world. The data suggested that 'crochet offers positive benefits for personal wellbeing with many respondents actively using crochet to manage mental health conditions and life events such as grief, chronic illness and pain'.[5] This aligns with how we've seen repetitive, sensory craft practices being so impactful in regulating the nervous system.

At the height of the Covid-19 pandemic, a study conducted with more than 1000 US participants who experienced anxiety found that 'gardening is one of many outdoor activities that has been shown to reduce the symptoms of anxiety and improve mental health'.[6] The impact of nature and trees on the brain and nervous system is well documented, and we know that even just looking at images of forests lowers the heart rate. Walking in nature has also been found to quickly lower stress levels, boost serotonin and create a sense of awe at the beauty of trees, sky and wildlife.[7] The benefits are even to be found in listening to birds singing! A 2022 study found that 'everyday encounters [of birdsong] were associated with time-lasting improvements in mental wellbeing ... not only in healthy people but also in those with a diagnosis of depression, the most common mental illness across the world'.[8]

The results of a pilot study on the impact of music interventions for people with depression found that listening to music significantly improved participants' mood and their associated symptoms, including sleep quality, quality of life and anhedonia (the reduced ability to experience pleasure).[9] Have you ever listened to a song so moving that it brings a sense of deep joy or happiness? A review of 28 music intervention trials identified music engagement as a 'natural antidepressant' that quickly produces dopamine, just as medication does.[10]

Dr Bruce Perry, an American clinical psychiatrist whose work focuses on children who've experienced trauma, has long championed the creative expression of rhythm. Perry highlights that rhythmic activities are an essential regulating tool for our psychological systems to be able to move into any kind of mainstream therapy. 'Patterned, repetitive and rhythmic somatosensory activity ... elicits a sensation of safety. Rhythm is regulating. All cultures have some form of patterned, repetitive rhythmic activity as part of their healing and mourning rituals – dancing, drumming, and davening (swaying slightly while reciting liturgical prayers).'[11]

There are also countless studies on the impact of dance in treating symptoms of post-traumatic stress disorder.[12] A study on choirs and singing found that this experience is the fastest way for a group of people to bond, and is being trialled in the United Kingdom as a key intervention for new mothers with postnatal depression.[13] Having met Lizzie in a small singing group in the months after my mother died, I personally attest to the benefits group singing offers for offsetting grief, despair and depression. And research has found that creative writing improves our immunity, an outcome that was tested on patients with HIV.[14]

I found a 2016 German study particularly astonishing. Participants with very limited art-making experience were asked to draw anything they liked for 45 minutes. It was discovered that they experienced a 15 per cent reduction in their cortisol levels (cortisol is that tricky hormone that activates our stress response).[15] Isn't this just a stunning finding – that just the act of making marks on a page interacts with our stress-hormone production?

And it's not just the making of art that can have positive impacts on our wellbeing – looking at it can provide health benefits, too. Dr Katherine Boydell, professor of mental health at the Black Dog Institute, Australia's leading research organisation for depression and mood disorders, has led arts-on-prescription research projects with amazing results. Of particular note is a collaboration with the Art Gallery of New South Wales called Culture Dose, which is described as 'an online art experience with your wellbeing as its primary focus'.[16] The program invited people to look at a series of artworks, and then answer questions about their emotional state afterwards.

Dr Boydell also created a body-mapping project that uses drawing as a group intervention tool. Boydell noted that 'after the eight-week program, we saw significant decreases in depression and loneliness, significant increases in a sense of community inclusion, and, of course, beautiful qualitative data like, "I can get through the week when I know I've got this Wednesday to look forward to." "I listened to music and sang in the car for the first time in years." Really powerful statements'.[17] This sounds familiar, and similar sentiments have been echoed in our eight-week workshops for ReMind.

Each of these studies came to the same conclusion: being involved in creative activities can help make us feel less alone, less anxious and less depressed. Instead, we feel more connected, more alive, more joyful, more capable of fun and delight and awe and wonder and friendship – the stuff of life! Creativity can indeed function as an antidepressant.

Over in the United Kingdom, it seems the social prescribing movement is picking up speed, with the global charitable foundation Wellcome Trust funding 'the largest study in the world bringing arts-based mental health interventions into a national health service'. Called the SHAPER Project (Scaling-up Health–Arts Programmes: Implementation and Effectiveness Research), the research, still in progress, will be the 'world's largest hybrid study on the impact of the arts on mental health embedded into a national healthcare system'.[18] Among the aims of the project, it acknowledges that while plenty of valuable research into the clinical impact of arts interventions on health exists, there hasn't been enough broad research to provide solutions for scalable interventions to be woven into primary health care, and that funding for these interventions is intermittent and undervalued. Tell me about it!

It seems that here in Australia, the healthcare system is still a while away from prescribing creativity to adults, but there is already a strong and compelling precedent for this in the world of caring for sick children.

Play is part of health

I happen to know someone who can speak about this deeply, someone with more than 20 years' experience. So I called up my dear friend Jono Brand. We met at uni back in the 1990s, kicking around in the same big gang of people doing student theatre in Brisbane. Jono was an accomplished actor and clown, side-splittingly funny to be with. After graduating, he got a job as Captain Starlight, a clown-character working in children's hospitals. I still remember when he got sent off to balloon-animal training. Today, Jono is the artistic director of the Captain Starlight program,[19] which has a presence in 12 major children's hospitals across Australia, a range of community-based programs in remote and regional areas, is one of the largest employers of performers in the country, and is part of Australia's most trusted charity. Jono explains a little more about his work:

The role of Captain Starlight is to turn up to play, and bring patients, families and staff into the play, if they want to. We do this because we know it really helps kids and their families feel supported, safe and reassured, and this shows up in evaluations of patients. We aren't there to meet therapeutic outcomes; we don't really know the details of what is going on for kids in the ward. We work alongside the clinical staff, but of course know our place, which is focusing on the wellbeing side of being sick, and in hospital, which can be really scary and traumatic for kids and their families.

We purposefully recruit people with live-performance experience, who can improvise and bring whatever is happening in the ward into the play, and use the character of the captain in that way. Captain Starlight is from another planet, and this is one of the fundamental pieces of the mythology that we drive home to our performers, so they can play up that naive, innocent clown, essentially. Pretending a teddy bear is a phone is funny and playful, but there's a real shift in status for that kid who's sitting in their bed. Suddenly, they have knowledge and expertise and it gives them more agency in a place where they are mostly powerless, to say, hey, actually, that's a teddy bear!

Our program goal is to positively reframe the hospital experience, which I love. And it can help strengthen the relationship that doctors and nurses have with patients too, if they join in the play. Our program evaluation shows that for every dollar spent on it, there is a $4.50 return in the community, in terms of improving longer-term health outcomes.

I read over a folder of evaluation reports and impact statements Jono sent me. A nursing manager said, 'Starlight is probably one of the most effective engagement tools that the hospital has ... If it wasn't there, I think we'd probably have more distressed consumers and I guess a symptom of distress is aggression as well.'[20] This nurse has landed on the crucial role of play in nervous system regulation, which is that it helps keep us grounded and able to respond from a place of calm rather than panic.

I imagine a program like this in all hospitals, not just children's ones. As Starlight's program motto says, happiness matters. It sure does. It matters for adults, too. When we need treatment, medicine and services. It matters that these experiences are designed in ways to also meet our psychological needs, which is so brilliantly the case for children and families through this program. It matters when folks who go to hospital for essential mental health treatment are traumatised by their lack of power in that environment.

Imagine some well-trained creative facilitators entering the ward to build rapport, trust and a sense of safety. Imagine if the soul-crushing fear that can come with having surgery, tests, chemotherapy or rehab treatment could be alleviated by embedding some creative practices into the healthcare system. Imagine! In times when we need to sleep well and have a regulated nervous system so that we can take in a lot of information about treatments and tests, creative prescribing could really impact the way patients present and then receive treatment.

The proof seems so clear, and completely accepted by the medical model when it comes to meeting children's needs, and so this very trusted, accepted approach could be extended to health care for adults, too. Right?

When did we decide that play was no longer a necessary feature of being – and staying – healthy once we become adults?

This sentiment is shared by Dr Christina Davies, a senior research fellow in the School of Allied Health at the University of Western Australia, whose research shows that two hours of arts participation a week improves mental health.[21] Her paper 'The Art of Being Healthy' describes a huge finding in the world of health promotion. Just like eating five servings of vegetables a day is good for our nutritional health, engaging in the arts, in some way, is good for our psychology. We knew it!

As Dr Davies explains, 'With sport, some people like to go to the park and kick around a ball, but then they go to a football game ... this should be the same with the arts. Do some colouring, do some painting, it doesn't matter if you're good or not good. And then, go to a gallery and see the works of a famous painter ... You don't have to be good at art for art to be good for you.'[22]

Creative play is in our nature

Remember when adult colouring books dominated every bestseller book list in the country, heck in half the world? The sudden obsession with this activity was a reminder that colouring, or even just exercising creativity, does something good for us – it's meditative, mindful and playful, and it can relax our busy brain. Studies showed that it reduces stress, fosters self-awareness and may improve anxiety, even with just ten minutes of colouring in.[23] And the only side effect was that you needed to sharpen your pencils more often. This moment in time revealed our human nature, that this pull to express ourselves in creative ways is hardwired into us. It's a ball of yarn that, if pulled and tugged at, unravels to reveal an even deeper, richer potential to harness innate human creativity to intentionally support our health.

For the past few years, I've facilitated Mental Health First Aid[24] training for hundreds of people across Australia. This training is designed for anyone – young or old – to learn skills in empathy and how to offer support to others.

I always ask attendees to introduce themselves by sharing something they do most days for their own mental health, something that helps keep them steady. And the answers? If I was a more organised person, perhaps past-me could have captured these responses, like data, to make this a little more oomphy. But a pie chart would look a little like this:

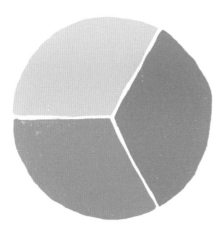

- 🔘 **33 per cent** spending time with pets (usually dogs)
- 🔘 **33 per cent** doing some kind of physical exercise (running, swimming, going to the gym)
- 🔘 **33 per cent** engaging in some kind of 'play' (playing music, dancing, journalling, gardening, knitting, painting, dressing up, sewing, building things, dressing up in medieval gear, whittling spoons, floral arranging, pole dancing, drag makeup, you name it).

Like the colouring books, these activities don't have to have a larger purpose. Instead, they act as the balm we need to soften the edges of life; to soothe anxious, busy minds; to carve out some solid ground beneath our feet when the world feels unsafe, unsteady and uncertain. (Global pandemic, anyone?) While seeing a therapist can be immensely helpful, we need to dedicate more than one hour of our week or fortnight to our mental health. Building a habit of doing things we enjoy can be a great way to do this.

Fun, nervous-system regulation and social connection are notably absent features of discussions in mainstream health about what's needed to repair and recover from poor mental health, and this is, in our view, a problematic omission.

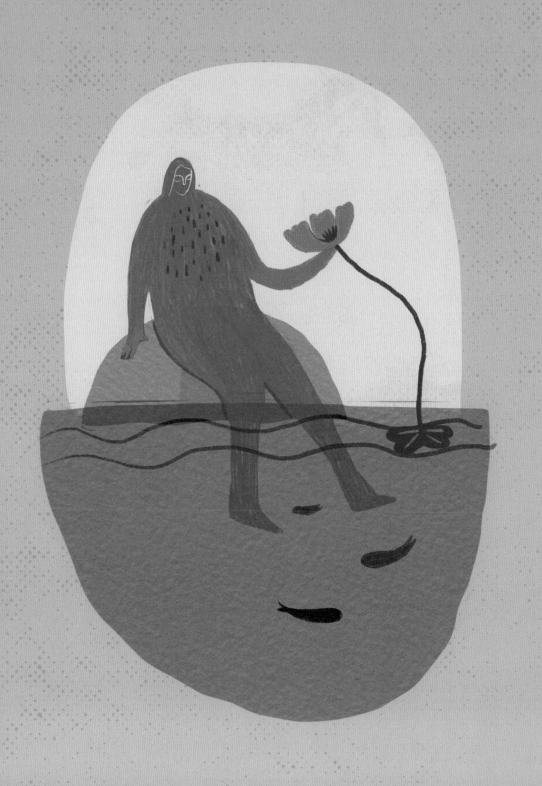

It's time to talk about mental health

We've made reference to mental health and mental wellbeing, and named particular, common experiences like depression, anxiety, trauma and PTSD. Let's take a closer look at what we mean.

One in five people in Australia and the United States, and one in four people in New Zealand and the United Kingdom, have what is considered to be a diagnosable mental health condition, the most common of these being anxiety then depression. It is estimated that 75 per cent of Australian adults have experienced a traumatic event in their life (although not everyone develops PTSD).[25]

At any time, around three in five people experience challenges to mental health.[26] Just like our physical health, where we may become rundown and have symptoms that get in the way of doing what we want to do, we may not have an illness per se, but we wouldn't describe ourselves as being well.

Sadly, we remain in this curious fantasy world where there is still shame in talking about our mental health, where 54 per cent of people with a diagnosable condition do not get professional support, and most people wait until things become really hard and tricky before doing anything at all.[27] At the same time, all the evidence tells us that the earlier we intervene – getting support, actively looking after our psychological wellbeing – the sooner and easier a return to health happens.

Mental health sits on a spectrum. Not every stressful event is traumatic. Not every worrying time becomes anxiety. But protecting your wellbeing is as important as supporting it when you experience illness. For people who live with, and through, periods of deep depression or debilitating anxiety, these can infuse every inch of life – relationships, work, study, physical health, living conditions, sense of identity. Understandably, it's an experience that leaves people wanting relief as quickly as possible. The symptoms themselves can cloud our sense of what we need and be at odds with what we want, and all up can make this road tricky, lonely and very much uphill.

Mental health:
the next pandemic?

Since December 2019, when most of the coast of New South Wales burned catastrophically – land scorched, millions of animals dead – it feels like the world has turned up the dial of Truly Intense Crap Going Down. In my little corner of the world, it's a relentless cascade, week after week, which seems to be, dare I say it, the new normal. I watch as people around my age (40s, 50s) start to unravel – health conditions, the slow burn of childhood trauma catching up, divorce, ageing parents, parenting and financial stress being the menu on offer. Pick one! Or pick three – all at once!

I watch as first-time parents crack under the weight of expectations to be perfect, in a culture that can lack support, childcare and that elusive village we need so much. Younger people have spent their fundamental years of development in isolation and lockdowns, the effect of which continues to show up in everyday life.

The cost of living and divided political climates make for an atmosphere of hysteria and anger, on social media anyway. Friends and I gather to commiserate about finding ourselves tasked with parenting kids in this weird and wonky time for the world, with so many unanswerable questions: Is the planet going to die? Will we all go to war about water? Are robots going to take over the world? Will there even be a future for me? There isn't a parenting book for this stuff.

The pandemic briefly suspended us in a moment of potential redefinition. Perhaps we might be able to redesign how much work consumes our lives. But the moment passed and now a global Gallup study has found we are more stressed than ever, and workplace wellbeing has stagnated since 2020.[28]

Geez. What a downer, huh?

Life can be pretty damn hard!

Not everyone who is affected by these life events has mental ill health. But it is no wonder that living with significant, challenging, chronic and debilitating mental health conditions is harder, and more common than ever.[29] No surprise that a 2020–21 report from the National Study of Mental Health and Wellbeing estimates that half of all young women in Australia experience anxiety and depression.[30] It feels like every week there's a new article shouting about the mental health epidemic.

New reports and statistics continue to paint an even more distressing picture for Indigenous Australians: suicide is the fifth leading cause of death, and one in four Aboriginal people live with a diagnosable mental health condition.[31] In 2023, Australian journalist and Wiradjuri man Stan Grant announced he was stepping back from television hosting due to the relentless racist abuse, hate speech and threats his family received. The intersection of colonisation, intergenerational trauma and public discourse means that to be Indigenous in this country will most certainly bring with it lived experiences of racism, discrimination, disadvantage and trauma.[32]

Transgender and non-binary identifying people are also four times as likely to experience mental health conditions, and LGBTQI identifying people are two and half times more likely.[33] Trans young people are also four times as likely to attempt suicide. This is at a time when the media is engaged in ongoing shouting matches about these identities, dehumanising trans people and reducing their lived experience to a political debate. Globally, one in three women experience sexual or physical violence,[34] one in five people with a disability report being discriminated against. Activists and advocates who champion these experiences on social media are so often the target of hate speech, death threats and cyber violence. These are all incredibly traumatic experiences to live through. I could go on.

I mention all these statistics because identity is a social experience that contributes to, and influences, our health. The way our culture affords or withholds privilege to people according to their race, class, gender, ability, sex and perceived vulnerability is an important piece of the puzzle in reflecting on why so many people experience mental health challenges.[35] The public conversations politicising people's identity and dehumanising their experience undoubtedly contributes to depletion of mental wellbeing.

Trauma research pinpoints that a lack of safety in being free to be oneself can contribute to an experience of trauma.[36] In essence, being seen and also valued are such intrinsic needs for our souls that not feeling these things wounds us. Deeply. That wound can show up in multiple ways, but very often as a sensation of deep fear and panic. As despair, hopelessness and feeling depressed. As anger, isolating us from those around us.

So it should come as no surprise that demand for psychology and other primary mental health services vastly exceeds supply.[37] Education in this field dutifully encourages the importance of seeking help, except that help is thin on the ground.

The point here is that life in these times can be pretty damn hard, y'all. Our psychological needs are difficult to meet in this state of play.

Do we have the answers?

Here in Australia, along with much of the Western world, mental ill health has long been (and still is) seen as a medical issue, one that can be treated – and is treated – with both medication and clinical therapy from either a psychiatrist or psychologist. Unlike a whole range of physical ailments and illnesses that can be diagnosed with a blood test or scan, diagnosing mental health conditions can be a little more elusive. And so, clinicians are guided by the DSM (Diagnostic and Statistical Manual of Mental Disorders), which is authored by the American Psychiatric Association and is currently in its fifth edition.

It's the field of psychiatry – doctors who specialise in psychiatric diagnosis and treatment – that determines the path for the acceptable way to treat conditions like depression, anxiety and PTSD. Curiously, what remains at the heart of this diagnostic tool, along with the treatment protocols, is the understanding that much of what is considered 'mental illness' is a brain-chemical imbalance, one that can be corrected or shifted with pharmaceutical medications such as antidepressants.

One in eight people are prescribed antidepressants in Australia, and 85 per cent of these are prescribed by GPs in five- to ten-minute appointments.[38] One in six people in the United Kingdom take antidepressants and these are so widely used that traces of them are found in Britain's drinking water.[39] Benzodiazepines (nervous system depressants for anxiety and insomnia) account for 40 per cent of pharmaceutical prescribing in the United States.[40]

These medications are intended and designed to increase the feel-good, mood-enhancer hormones in the brain, such as serotonin and noradrenaline. You can tell that the medications are working if the people taking them notice an increase in energy, and perhaps improved sleeping and appetite, as well as overall enhanced mood. For some people, this is exactly what happens, which is wonderful.

Except that, and this is huge, really: the brain-chemical imbalance theory is not proven.[41] Yep. There are many studies and study reviews[42] that reach similar conclusions. The best we currently have is the shared agreement that 'depression is probably not caused by brain-chemical imbalance', yet the treatment remains unchanged. It's important to say that adjustments to our brain chemistry can definitely impact and improve our mood. But this means that medication is treating a symptom and not the cause. Not only that, but for many people, the side effects of taking antidepressants can often mimic the exact conditions they are trying to improve – increased anxiety, insomnia, agitation, nausea, fatigue and feeling numb.[43]

How does this happen? It's a curious situation given we are living in a time when having evidenced-based treatment is insisted upon. And yet, contrastingly, social and creative prescribing, which works wonders for loads of the people engaged in these small, scattered initiatives, many of which have very robust and convincing evaluation reports, repeatedly struggles for funding and credibility due to an apparent lack of evidence.

Dr Jon Jureidini, a child psychiatrist based in Adelaide, points out in his 2020 book with Leemon McHenry *The Illusion of Evidence-Based Medicine: Exposing the crisis of credibility in clinical research*[44] that drug companies are known to fund huge-scale studies with vast numbers of people as a way to ensure significant results. However, Dr Jureidini believes that 'if you can show something in a small study [that] stands out, then that's much more likely to be meaningful than something that you need a meta-analysis of 15 different studies to show a fractional benefit'.[45]

If the world advertised a vacancy for the role of a treatment for depression, would the pills get the job? Is it time to look at the selection criteria again, and make sure we haven't discounted some other really good applicants? Or maybe we need a team, with a diverse set of skills and attributes? Medication – sure – but also equally valuable, perhaps listening to music? Or connecting with nature? Or skating with a group of roller derby chicks who get you slicing up a rink and make you feel truly alive?

Is it medicine we need?

Medicine is, in its truest sense, something to make life feel better. It lessens pain. It makes infections subside. It makes a functional, active life possible. Except, not always. Tragically, and in many people's view unnecessarily, medicine too often fails in improving symptoms for those with chronic pain and poor mental health.

Judging by their name – antidepressants – we would presume, and rightly so, that the purpose of these medications is to counter the sometimes-debilitating experiences of feeling depressed, despairing, anxious and in grief. To anti the depress. To up the down. To light the dark and reduce distress. But what if the definition of antidepressant wasn't just a prescribed, regulated pharmaceutical, but any form of proven, consistent course of action that is safe, accessible and performs the job of lifting one's mood, generally improving energy, sleep and appetite, and overall feelings of wellbeing?

What if our health system prescribed social activities for people who felt lonely, instead of, or even as well as, prescribing Zoloft? Or prescribed walking in nature for overwhelmed, anxious and overworked people? The effects and also side effects would be far more palatable. This is essentially what social and creative prescribing aims to do. As British–Swiss journalist Johann Hari says in his bestselling book *Lost Connections: Why you're depressed and how to find hope*, 'What if changing the way we live – in specific, targeted, evidence-based ways – could be seen as an antidepressant too?'[46]

Lighting the lanterns

For many people, taking medication is the crucial difference between being okay and being so very not okay. For the many people possibly reading this who use antidepressants, this can be hard to digest. This is not an effort to denounce the use of pharmaceutical antidepressants. If this treatment helps you, that is a real truth that can exist alongside the fact that we have a system that overprescribes them,[47] and seems to lack other options. In a nutshell, this isn't necessarily the solution for everyone.

Dr Mark Melek, an Australian practising GP and advocate of holistic medicine, says that sometimes the use of medication for mental health issues just creates some breathing room, some space for people to explore and engage in the things that will continue to be really helpful in the long term. This isn't an either/or scenario. What works for one person might not work for another. Furthermore, many antidepressants and anxiety medication are intended for short-term use, not years and decades.

If pills aren't your jam, what about some of the other things that might do the job in a different way? In fact, more and more studies are revealing that depression and anxiety are often caused by experiencing trauma, which actually responds far better to embodied, somatic treatments such as movement therapy; yoga; EMDR (eye movement desensitisation and reprocessing), a psychotherapy treatment that reduces distressing feelings by using bilateral stimulation; and neurofeedback, a non-invasive therapy that teaches people how to consciously control their brainwaves.[48]

There is also plenty of evidence suggesting that social and systemic circumstances and experiences can lead to depression, anxiety and activated trauma responses. A 'biopsychosocial'[49] model of mental health acknowledges the link between biology, psychology and also social factors – whether someone experiences poverty, racism or an absence of opportunity. It's now keenly understood that if you have a high rating on the Adverse Childhood Experiences (ACE) scale, you are also more likely to experience depression or anxiety in your lifetime.[50] In my social-work-trained brain, this has always seemed darn obvious to me.

There's a vast spectrum of 'non-clinical interventions' (i.e. anything outside of the medical modalities of medication and prescribed psychiatric or psychological therapies) that can provide an increased sense of self-worth, connection to others, improved energy, and experience of pleasure. One of those interventions? You guessed it, creative practice! (Along with physical exercise, meditation, mindfulness, somatic therapies, volunteering and community participation.)

So to recap: science and evidence are essential to our lives. We need science for life-saving medicine and certainly for acute conditions when there's no clear alternative. We also need agency and control over our life and to recognise that while medication can help us, it isn't the be-all and end-all of mental health treatment. It's still worth keeping the door open to the possibility of new ideas, approaches, treatments and offerings that can work in tandem with medicine and pharmacology.

Psychological therapy is a fantastic, helpful intervention for so many people and part of the pathway for dealing with these mental health challenges. This service system isn't without its problems, though. As Vanessa Edwige, psychologist and chair of the Australian Indigenous Psychology Association said in our chat over Zoom, 'People who have experienced trauma or adverse events often find it difficult to engage in talking therapies. Focusing on developing the skills of self-regulation enables them to engage in the therapeutic process. We need widespread community education for people to understand how they themselves can have a sense of control over their nervous system and how this is key to de-escalating trauma responses. This enables a sense of agency and empowerment around their own wellbeing.'

The medical model asks us to be fairly passive and at the mercy of this treatment system. In times when we are most overwhelmed, most incapacitated, most dysregulated, we suddenly need to navigate referral pathways and assessment criteria and we are told to wait our turn. The support system itself creates an alarming dynamic of disempowerment, and helplessness in the help-seeking process. For people already feeling a lack of control in their life, this seems truly the worst outcome of a system designed to help, not hinder. Of course, many people who do seek help get it, and a lot of that help is enormously beneficial. But at its worst? This system can be traumatising.

With an overextended system alongside lots of treatment experiences that don't quite meet most people's actual needs, we then have a community desperate to find their own answers, wherever they can. When people become deflated and distrusting of the medical treatment path for

Building the body of
evidence for the role
of creative practices in
health treatments is
a little like searching
for small lanterns
across the land.

—

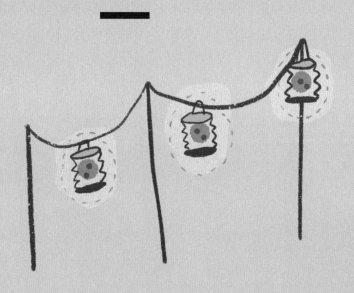

depression or PTSD, there's a risk of reliance on coping strategies such as substance use, or unvetted, unqualified life coaches, or the hectic stream of 'wellbeing' and life-improvement content on social media.

Working in this area it feels as though we are in a necessary transition that demands a broadening of what we offer when people - heck, when whole communities - are brought to their knees with the shudders of despair, the panic of fear and anxiety, and the chaotic ways these experiences shatter our connection to ourselves and each other.

So, what's the alternative?

In place of the brain-chemical model of mental illness, there is another school of thought that a growing number of clinicians, therapists and researchers support: mental ill health is the result of psychological needs, such as community, purpose, safety and self-worth, not being met. And all of this is influenced by the systems and social structures that we live within.

Sickness can be more than just a collection of cells and chemicals, it can be a complex experience influenced by, and sometimes caused by, the world we inhabit. Where we happen to sit on the wheel of privilege and power matters a great deal when it comes to our health. Researchers know without a doubt that how lonely you are, how poor you are and how psychologically 'well' you are will greatly inform your overall health.[51]

Poverty, loneliness, violence, discrimination, intergenerational trauma and unemployment are considered to be social determinants of health, meaning that each of these factors plays a large role in how we see ourselves, thus how we feel, and how we move through the world. It makes sense that losing a job, not having enough money to eat or buy new shoes, and being isolated would make you feel depressed. While this is oversimplifying, it's a little strange that someone experiencing those things is offered medication instead of a job, new shoes or a chance to make friends.

Dr Gabor Maté, internationally acclaimed Hungarian-Canadian physician, writer and thought leader in trauma, addiction and childhood health, has described in great detail the body-mind unity concept that many clinical and medical practitioners are beginning to build into their treatment.[52]

A 2015 paper on this theory says that body-mind unity in health isn't denying the biomedical approach to health, but expanding it to incorporate 'psychological and eco-social factors as a strong impact for health and disease'. Essentially, our psychology influences our physical health, and so does the environment and society we live in.[53] Dr Maté acknowledges that many other cultures already understand this, and these traditional ways of treating illness have been discredited historically by Western medicine.[54]

There is a new field of study that Dr Maté describes in his book *The Myth of Normal: Trauma, illness and healing in a toxic culture*, called psychoneuroimmunology (or PNI for short), which maps the links between our brain and body, nervous system, pain receptors and hormones. Rather than treating these things as separate, PNI requires us to look at them holistically, as connected systems. The book includes numerous accounts of patients presenting with physical symptoms or conditions, only to be relieved by treating childhood trauma, or finding undeniable links between their experience of racism or poverty and the illness they develop.

I am reminded of a profound and ultimately life-changing moment I experienced when I was 22. I was a newly minted social worker with two jobs: one at a rape crisis centre and sexual assault helpline, and the other in a young women's housing and sexual assault service. It was increasingly stressful supporting women – who themselves were often struggling with addiction and PTSD – who were trying to flee physical, emotional and sexual violence.

A few years into this work I began experiencing a constant, dull feeling of pressure in my chest and shortness of breath, all day, every day. I was young and otherwise pretty fit. At the same time, I became more withdrawn from my social life and stopped sleeping well, suffering from intense nightmares. I would cry a lot, sometimes at nothing and then at everything. I felt like I was fighting an invisible war, a war against women and children that no-one seemed to care that much about. The chest pains intensified. They were scary, and very, very unusual.

I went to see a GP and spent 24 hours on a heart monitor, which revealed absolutely nothing. I got blood tests and was told I had dangerously high cholesterol, something that would require taking medication for the rest of my life. It was also suggested I try a range of medications – from antidepressants to anti-anxiety pills, sleeping tablets and others I couldn't even pronounce. A gut instinct told me this wasn't the solution, despite my need for answers. After seeing multiple specialists, all of whom seemed to show little curiosity about anything other than the physical symptoms I was experiencing, nothing changed. Finally, a friend suggested I see a different GP, who was also a doctor of traditional Chinese medicine.

He asked me a lot of questions about what I did and how I managed such stressful work, especially for someone so young. 'Oh, I have boundaries,' I said, parroting the standard line that social workers are taught. He looked at me and said, 'Your heart is hurting. You are carrying the pain of these women like it is your pain. This is not your pain to carry.'

It was the best thing he could have said to me. My good fortune in seeing a doctor of Chinese medicine, unbeknown to me at the time, was that this school of medicine, one of the most ancient in existence, views emotions and physical health as inextricably connected, influencing each other in a feedback loop.[55]

The exposure to trauma stories, day after day at work, was unconsciously interacting with my psychology, triggering a pretty significant vicarious trauma response. This manifested in multiple physical symptoms, affecting my nervous system, hormones, mind, brain and heart.

I took leave from work and spent the next couple of months applying what I see now as creative first aid. I played the piano. I drew. I listened to music. I spent time at the beach. The chest pains disappeared. Repeat tests showed my cholesterol had magically dropped. I stopped crying so much – not that there's anything wrong with crying, but crying while buying cat food had started to feel a little awkward.

I also saw a clinical psychologist. I learnt about vicarious trauma and how it manifests and why. With a bit of distance and support, I realised how much this work was impacting me, and that I needed to rebalance things before I lost myself entirely. I handed in my resignation and flew to the other side of the world to live in Scotland.

Creative First Aid

Taking control: protecting our own mental health

The point here is this: our mental and psychological wellbeing is influenced by what is happening in our lives, and also the presence, or absence, of things such as family, community, financial security, employment. This in turn influences our internal psychology via our nervous system. Managing our mental health can't always change the challenges of life. But what we can do, and be empowered to do, is understand the way our nervous system, our body and our psychological needs interact, and how those systems behave when under pressure and threat. We can learn how we can send messages to those systems that will keep us in a space of regulated, grounded calm as much as possible, so we can navigate rocky roads.

Being in tune with our bodies and understanding our own psychological responses gives us agency when interacting with the health system. Creative first aid offers a path to this inner wisdom. We don't need to be passive recipients of treatments we don't fully understand. We can ask questions, advocate for ourselves and listen to that tiny voice telling us something isn't quite right, even if doctors are saying that everything is fine.

I lost my mother to a rare cancer that first manifested as an annoying, persistent cough. Her determination to trust her gut that something was amiss ultimately led to the diagnosis of that lurking, hidden disease. The legacy of that loss is often in my own mind when pursuing answers to health stuff. Yes, trust doctors, but also, trust yourself.

Sickness isn't just cells and bacteria. It's also social and political systems influencing and interacting with our psychology. This means that the suite of treatment offerings for people experiencing psychological challenges needs to encompass medical, social and environmental interventions. See a psychologist – this is such a fantastic and helpful process for so many people. Try and take medications – if they work for you. Equally important? Connecting to enjoyment of life, to other people, to moments of awe, joy and wonder. And it's here that creative first aid steps onto the stage.

Creativity as medicine: a prescribed dose of joy and play

It was deathly quiet on the Zoom call, where close to 60 people had assembled for MakeShift's four-week Press Play course in the wintery months of deep lockdown for many. Lots of people shared that they were dealing with daily symptoms of depression, anxiety, complete overwhelm and burnout. Getting out of bed was hard, and it was a miracle they were even on this call.

Helena Fox, an award-winning author, was our facilitator. She set our group the task of writing for ten minutes from a prompt – an image of a tree. We had just heard her talk about the way that writing can be a profound act of self-care – of release, reflection, curiosity, connection, communication and play. Helena asked if anyone wanted to share. They read beautiful, imaginative little stories. Silly, nonsensical, moving, playful, serious, comedic, sensory – it was all there. There was surprise, generally. Exclamations about how calm people felt, how relaxed, how different. Something had... shifted.

'I feel like I've just had a three-hour nap,' one person wrote as the workshop wrapped up. 'It's like it just poured out of me. I had no idea I would be able to write anything, or even have anything to say. I am shocked!' wrote another. 'So surprised at the writing exercise. Just ten minutes and I felt entirely different, awake, inspired. It was fun, and that was the most surprising thing about it,' someone chimed in.

'This is the way that writing can be an act of release, of play,' explained Helena. 'We can take words out for a walk. We can make anything happen, anything in the world, on a page. We are completely in control.' The act of writing can help clear out our thoughts, kind of like dragging and dropping files into the digital recycling bin. In fact, expressive writing, even for just 15 minutes a day, has been proven to foster improvements in both physical and psychological wellbeing.[56]

Taking a tablet requires trust. We can't necessarily feel or notice the effect as it is happening, but later reflect (hopefully): 'Oh, I do feel a bit better.' In the same way, intentionally prescribing ourselves a practice of creativity for medicinal purposes requires a leap of faith at first. We might not instantly notice the impact, but we must trust in the body of evidence telling us that many people who tried this have found improvements to their mood, sense of self, and ability to connect and make decisions based on logic and reason.

Having a doctor prescribe this to us might happen in the future, but for now, we can begin ourselves. In Chapter 4, we take you through how to understand your own nervous system, and what it needs. And then in Chapter 5 we introduce the Creative Dispensary – 50 creative prescriptions designed to act medicinally to influence the way we feel.

The outcomes from using creativity as a type of medicine? We actively learn to regulate our nervous system, which is key to our wellbeing. We create space to find meaning beyond our inner world. We get to practise trying new things, making mistakes, being curious, taking risks. We slowly connect to glimmers of joy, delight, gratitude, awe and wonder. Through these habits, we prime ourselves to connect with others, and grow our deep wisdom about ourselves.

Creative first aid vs art therapy: what's the difference?

It's understandable to think these two things are the same, so I want to make an important distinction here between creative first aid and art therapy.

Art therapy is a really fantastic and useful discipline that incorporates creative methods of expression to work through therapeutic goals. It is a style of clinical treatment done by a therapist, guiding, supervising and helping someone reflect in the way that traditional therapy does. Art therapists undertake significant training to deliver this to people in a clinical setting. An example might be exploring traumatic childhood memories using expressive journalling and painting.

By contrast, creative first aid is about engaging in creativity because it makes us feel good. Rather than being guided by therapists, we can learn from artists and creatives. It is something that any person is capable of doing, in their own time, just as we could join a community sports team – for fun, social connection, for those feel-good endorphins. We could also see a sports therapist – to improve our mindset, technique, manage injury and stress relating to playing. They are two entirely different processes, both valuable.

Loads of the studies that report the positive outcomes of engaging with creativity use the term 'art therapy' to describe engaging in any creative activity that has health benefits. This again speaks to the absence of a shared language for talking about these approaches, and the fact that there is a fundamental difference between engaging in therapy that uses art interventions, and engaging in art activities because they are enjoyable, and happen to also have health benefits.

The exciting future of creative and social prescribing

In 2019, the National Health Service (NHS) in the UK committed five million pounds in funding to establish a national social prescribing academy.[57] This development has already provided life-affirming support to thousands of community members, but also relieved a very over-stretched health system in many cases where a referral to a community garden, local choir or art class in lieu of a service waiting list means that those with the most urgent and acute needs are able to receive therapeutic treatment sooner. This is an exciting advance in the progress of creative and social prescribing being woven into primary health care.

In 2022, MakeShift participated in a summit by Creative Australia that culminated in 'Connected Lives: Creative Solutions to the Mental Health Crisis', a report that outlines a series of recommendations for government and identifies ways that arts interventions in health care could be funded.

We at MakeShift conducted our own pilot test of prescribing creativity as a health intervention in late October 2022. We set up our Creative Clinic out of a shipping container in the CBD centre, dispensing doses of creativity as an antidote for living through a pandemic. We treated nurses, psychologists, cancer patients, psychiatric patients, the local mayor, corporate workers, council workers and weary individuals looking to ease their tender nervous system, all of whom turned up for their pre-booked 30-minute appointment.

The clinic comprised of five intervention rooms, each staffed by our team of Creative Clinicians wearing green boiler suits. Patients entered with an intake question: 'Do you have a history of dressing up – does it run in your family?' Tentative people quickly softened into wide-eyed laughter when issued with a wig, sparkly glasses, a swishy cape, a top hat. Next, people sat in front of a coloured mirror and drew their own portrait (blind!). Almost impossible to do this without laughing – an instant endorphin boost.

Then it was into Thread Therapy – a comfy space with giant cushions and a big bowl of coloured beads. The act of choosing, threading and repetitive making was a catalyst for rest and slowing down busy brains. Next, patients stepped into a mini living forest – an immersive experience of plants to smell and touch, along with headphones playing bird calls, running water and nature sounds to help take urban dwellers into nature.

The appointment ended in the Observation Room, where disco balls hung from trees and weird sunglasses were given to participants to wear for a few minutes in order to let the dose settle in, check for side-effects and to see the world through a new lens.

'I just feel completely alive. Full of joy.' This was a common post-dose comment, along with others that often moved us to tears: 'I was anxious, and now I'm calm'; 'I felt nervous, and now so relaxed'; 'I came in so busy, and now? I feel human again.'

Our comrade in creative prescribing, Jill Bennett, heads The Big Anxiety, a festival programmed in partnership with the University of New South Wales that combines arts interventions with mental health conversations and support. The festival aims to 'reposition mental health as a collective, cultural responsibility, rather than simply a medical issue'.[58]

Things are certainly happening. Our dream is that we normalise being creative, and the act of doing creative things, for everyone, in every neighbourhood. Perhaps in another decade's time it will be completely normal to go to your GP and walk out with a referral to a psychologist, a walking group and a life drawing class. Maybe our Creative Clinic will be installed in health hubs and hospitals across the country. These little beginnings are growing, and have the potential to transform the way we meet, approach and support the vast majority of us who encounter really tough times just living in our body and mind. We all deserve peace, joy and connection.

❋ **Field note** – The unexpected remedy of floristry: Jenita's story

We first met Jenita at one of our eight-week ReMind programs in 2021. Here's her story.

'To start with, I was very sick and, well, we just didn't know why. I was a town planner at the time, doing 60 hours a week. My life was chaos, absolute chaos, and my anxiety levels were really high. My early diagnosis, before I knew I had a brain tumour, was severe anxiety and severe mental health issues. I ended up in a facility for a little while, because I had a bit of a breakdown. But my symptoms didn't get any better.

'My psychiatrist suggested that before increasing medication again, I get some tests done just to check there was nothing organic going on. I got an appointment the next day for an MRI. My life changed forever after that. They'd found a tumour on my brain. They gave me ten days to live from when they found it, but then they were able to reduce it with really strong steroids, which saved my life. It was really hard to fathom. I felt like I had this thing in my body that I needed to get rid of, like a splinter or something foreign, but I knew I couldn't.

'So to cope, I thought, "I'm going to name this tumour, I'm going to give it a name and get to know it and I'm going to say my goodbyes over the next ten days and that's

how I'm going to do this." I had my own rules. I gave it a name and that helped me. Its name is Charlie.

'When I landed in the ReMind program, I thought that creativity was such a luxury that I just couldn't afford. I felt like I didn't have any extra time for something like creativity. "I can't be doing this!" I'd say to myself. But I stayed in the program and every week I began to look forward to these really beautiful, peaceful couple of hours. It really just turned things around for me. I've got goosebumps and tears just thinking about it.

'Creative time became necessary for processing how I handled living with the tumour and for managing all the many care systems I had in place. I made creativity a part of my care plan. I told my support workers that this practice is as essential as any of my neuro appointments.

'When I first discovered MakeShift, my life was probably 10 per cent creative and 90 per cent admin and task related, but now it has flipped. My life is full of creativity now. I love it so much. I feel 'myself' and more human when I'm creative. It's like now I have permission to be creative. I can see the importance of it – and it is so good for my anxiety. To be honest, MakeShift saved my life.

'I'd been a member of a floristry club for ten years, but then a floristry course kind of turned up in my life and I enrolled. I was really nervous, but I gave myself permission to try it and it's changed my life more than I ever expected. Flowers are so calming for me; they have become my medicine.

'Now I seek out creativity wherever I can – it is leading me to the person I want to be. Everything is getting a little bit easier every day and the flowers smell so nice!'

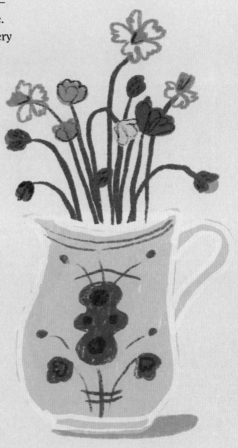

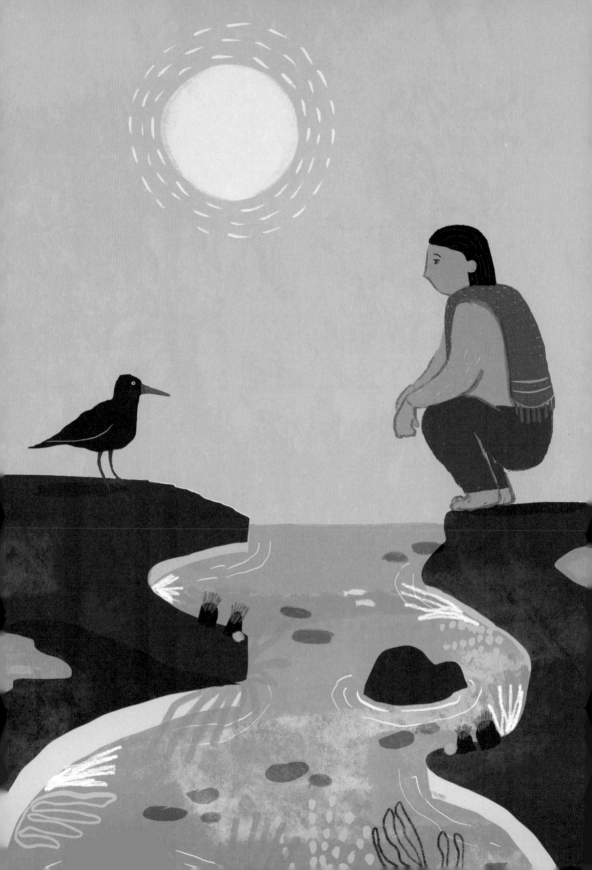

CHAPTER 3

Human Kind: How the outside world can help us grow our inside world

by Lizzie

In the last chapter, we learnt about the ways creativity can act like medicine, influencing the internal chemistry of our brains and hormones, and shifting the way our nervous system responds to periods of intense depression or anxiety. This chapter focuses on three vital parts of human life, outside of our bodies and minds, that have a two-way relationship with creativity: joy, nature and community. These things are closer to us when we are also engaged with our own creativity, and the more we connect with them, the deeper the pool of creativity inside us becomes.

We often need to work hard for these vital elements of human life. Our capitalist, productivity-led society that promotes busyness and consumption can make the path to access joy, to connect with nature, and to find community difficult, so it takes a bit of creativity to reach them. But once we find them, they in turn strengthen our capacity to be creative.

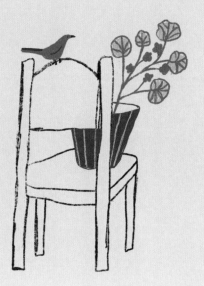

'Rather than cursing the darkness, what if we planted some seeds?'

Ross Gay[1]

1. Joy

Joy begins with glimmers

On the white brick walls of our office, written in Posca pen on a piece of card, are the words: *A creative habit can transform lives.* This is one of the underlying principles of our work at MakeShift and something that I have witnessed personally, as lead facilitator of our ReMind program. Next to this card is another important reminder: *Don't forget the glimmers!* I look to this reminder frequently and apply it as though it were MakeShift's mission statement.

So what is a glimmer? The psychological use of the word 'glimmer'[2] was first suggested by clinician Deb Dana in 2018, who described it as something small, fleeting and marvellous. The opposite of a glimmer is a trigger, something that brings about feelings of danger, of being unsafe or under threat. Glimmer hunting is harnessing something that you find delightful, like a corporate commuter in their own silent disco at the bus stop, or green moss on smooth rocks (it's different for everyone), to cue the nervous system towards a state of safety, where you can experience mindfulness, curiosity and joy. Glimmers, therefore, can be a very meaningful antidote to feelings that arise from a trigger. It's important to mention here that bringing attention to glimmers doesn't dissolve the suffering we experience with triggers. But they can remind us that wellbeing isn't simply the absence of difficult feelings, it is also about the presence of good ones.

For example, if you find a glimmer, a message gets sent to your nervous system that indicates you are safe. With this tide of safety comes a felt sense of balance or regulation, and the possibility of connection, which then cues a deep feeling of pleasure that stems from joy. Glimmers don't guarantee joy, but they are a portal to get us there.

The word glimmer makes me think of a subtle-coloured rainbow that you might find on an early morning frosticle (frosty icicle) in winter. Something that is elusive, easy to miss and fleeting, but if you catch it, it can light you up from the inside. Glimmers can pop up organically throughout the day, or we can cultivate them.

Sounds a bit like magic, right? Feels a bit like it too, but there's neuroscience to back this up. Finding a glimmer activates one of the most important nerves in our body, one that controls and regulates our emotional response. The vagus nerve is somewhat like the superhighway of the body, sending vital information between our brain and internal organs, including our gut. Experiencing a glimmer is the feeling of our biology being in a place of connection or regulation. It's the soothing feeling of a long, slow, involuntary sigh.

Glimmers are my go-to, and hunting them has been a lifelong creative habit. They can be hard to find when I'm feeling wonky, but like tiny anchors they keep me grounded when life tries to tug out my roots.

For more than a decade now, my role in MakeShift has been to work with artists of all different mediums to bring creativity and connection to people experiencing mental health symptoms.

In working with a wide range of people with PTSD and complex PTSD,[3] it has been impossible not to bear witness to the cracks in our current mental health treatment model, where a distinct sense of disconnection prevails. Over and over, people have joined our programs desperately seeking a way to reconnect to themselves and to the world around them, to find a sense of belonging. Applying creativity has been a fundamental tool that has enabled this to happen, and the process begins by noticing glimmers.

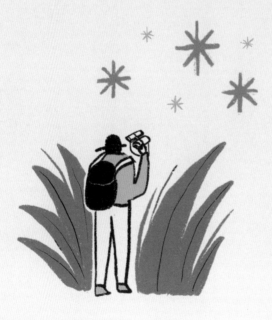

✳ **Field note** – Stargazing in police boots: Kate's story

Let's meet Kate. She looked to the stars as glimmers while working in a high-pressure, stressful environment with the federal police. Kate was in the police force for 30 years. During that time, she was a general duties cop and a first responder to murders, suicides and domestic violence cases. I spoke with Kate three years after she completed one of our ReMind programs. When we first began chatting, she sounded tired, but pepped up when the conversation moved towards music.

'I had never played a musical instrument until MakeShift sent me a ukulele in the post. When I did the ReMind program, life was very blurry. I was at rock bottom, really low. One day I went out for coffee and then when I came home there was a big box on the doorstep. Honestly, I was like a kid in a toyshop unpacking that box. It all started from that day, things shifting for me. It gave me something to focus on straight away.

'The ukulele is what struck me the most, and learning to play it on Zoom that week, I guess that really opened a door for me. I couldn't really play it, but since it came in that box, I have kept it up and now I'm in a little group. I'd never touched an instrument before I got sent one, and now I play Peter, Paul and Mary songs – "The Marvelous Toy", I love that one! It keeps me engaged, takes me back to nice places, nice memories through songs from my past, and it quietens down the anxiety. I go out every week and play in this local group and I really like it. It brings me some joy, which I needed because I was really stuck. Some days are harder than others, but now my husband just tells me to go and play my ukulele if I'm having a tough day. I wish I had the ukulele when I was in the muster room.

'The muster room is the main room where the radio is, where the calls come in. It's up really loud and there's constant updates and call-outs to different areas for different cases. You're on high alert sitting in that room, eating lollies and drinking coffee to stay awake. I did like the 3 am shift, though. I'd go outside, look up and see the stars and it was so quiet, like being given an instant dose of calm. I still love that time of night when the world is asleep. It's the tiny things that help. Like a billion stars can really remind you of your place in the world. I don't know, it just really helps to stop and look up at the sky in the quiet of the night sometimes, as a way to catch your breath. I think it is something I will do forever.'

I imagine Kate in full uniform, standing in polished boots outside the police station she has been assigned to. I can see her head upward facing, drinking in starlight as a momentary reprieve from the fast, wired pace of the muster room. It is within the dark sky spaces that Kate seeks solace.

Joy, an invitation to health

Joy! It's a musical word, but not just one you find in worship songs. The neurobiology of joy is complex, with four neurotransmitters (messengers) in the brain that promote positive feelings: dopamine, serotonin, oxytocin and endorphins. These four feel-good chemicals are essential for humans to experience, as often as possible – a free, readily available natural antidepressant. Their levels ebb and flow with our mood and interactions with the world. Sometimes we need to work hard at tweaking the ratio of these four hormones in our body. Through curiosity and play, we can open up the portal to experiencing joy, delight and wonder.

It seems a cruel tension that a salve for pain – physical, psychological, spiritual – might be joy, yet in these difficult states of pain, the feeling can seem miles away, unreachable. What we do know is that joy rarely sits in the same giant mixing bowl as self-criticism or judgement. It is a moment when we are briefly outside ourselves, forgetting our worries and thoughts even, just elevated by something wondrous that takes our focus. This means the fleeting nature of joy can co-exist in the very same bowl as pain, grief and loss. Like the time my dog came to check on me, resting her head and looking at me tenderly with her deep-brown eyes and freckled nose, then promptly sneezing in my face while I was in a moment of tears.

Ross Gay, an American poet and the author of *Inciting Joy*, talks powerfully about joy, nature connection and having community as a human right, and how being deprived of these plentiful things is a disprivilege. He goes on to say, 'life, though it is a gift, is not a privilege ... What would happen if we acknowledged that none of this (joy, community) is privilege, but rather as it should and could be? And what if we figured out, together, in a million different ways, how to make it so?'[4] Joy, nature and community belong to everyone.

In her memoir, *Nothing Bad Ever Happens Here*, Australian author Heather Rose talks about living with chronic arthritis, which causes her excruciating and debilitating pain. She speaks of pain as a gateway into other places, and into the world of creativity. 'Joy is my daily practice. Joy is my discipline. Joy is as essential as food, water, any diet, supplement or regime. Joy is an invitation to health. Joy is flow,' she says.

Joy can be found even in our darkest moments, and the more we actively practise seeking joy, the more we benefit from it. Joy and happiness are often used interchangeably. However, happiness technically refers to the pleasurable feelings (emotions) that result from a situation, an experience or objects, whereas joy is a state of mind that can be found even in times of grief or uncertainty.[5]

Research shows that daily experiences of awe, curiosity, gratitude, love and joy can put the average person on a trajectory of growth, success and positive social connection, and can also prevent those who are suffering from following a downward spiral.[6] Instead of joy being tucked away as a luxury of a privileged few – those with time and money and the absence of illness, pain or poverty – more and more it's being recognised as a fundamental human right.

Let us then see joy as a requirement, a non-negotiable dosage of wonder for life and being alive. And if it is thin on the ground, then we can actively cultivate it through creative practices and habits. We can prescribe joy for ourselves, while we also continue to advocate that joy be prescribed by clinicians. As our friend, writer Helena Fox declared, 'Play is a moment to recharge our joy molecules!'

Maybe we need a new word, as joy is so wholly tied up with a perception of trouble-free happiness. *Duende* in Spanish is vaguely translated as an enhanced sense of emotion, heart and expression. Tied to the experience of hearing flamenco music, it's defined as 'what gives you chills, makes you smile or cry as a bodily reaction to an artistic performance that is particularly expressive', and comes from a people whose culture is enriched by diaspora and hardship, the human condition of joys and sorrows.[7]

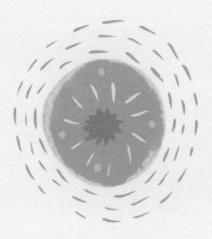

Imagination

It is 2023 and Dr Bessel van der Kolk, psychiatrist, researcher and author of the bestselling book *The Body Keeps the Score*, is running a two-day workshop about trauma from a windowless conference theatre. It's in the basement of a large city building and I'm there with 600 others under fluorescent lights, squished like peas in rows of chairs. The irony of the content we are there to learn being delivered in a space so uninformed of trauma! My first instinct is to run (it's one of my trauma symptoms). I sit down, feel fidgety, notice my heart rate increasing. I become flooded with a primal feeling to flee, so I check for the doors. This response to being shut up in a large space with no windows is 'normal' for me, so I work hard to find a glimmer to anchor myself and override the need to leap out of my chair and bolt. I take off my shoes and do a five-second reboot – ask myself, *What can I hear, see, smell, feel, touch?* My breath starts to slow. I look up at the very high ceiling and in the corner there is light refracting from the technical equipment on stage, making a flickering pattern. It is a little like what sunlight does on water when it glistens. I feel calmer.

Dr van der Kolk talks about purpose being the fundamental tool for self-regulation. It's the thing that can help us gain balance within our nervous system. He tells us that just like earthworms moving through soil from one place to the next, purpose is the pure energy to do something or to get somewhere. It is a powerful motivating force that resides within all of us and one of the ways to unlock this powerful human instinct of motivation is through the activation of pleasure and finding joy. Dr van der Kolk explains that experiencing pleasure makes us feel good, competent and capable. It gives us a sense of agency, power and belonging, and is critical in any therapy.

'We are all fundamentally mystical creatures,' Dr van der Kolk explains, 'that get pleasure from being in sync with others. It is very important that we establish a sense of connection to ourselves and others around us and to the environment, and heal in this state of synchronicity. It is what opens up possibilities and our imagination.'[8]

The word imagination lands on me gently, like a fallen feather. *Like birds,* I think to myself, *our imagination cannot be contained, it knows no borders.* There is a tremendous freedom that comes with hearing Dr van der Kolk lead this discussion about imagination, and I'm reminded of a conversation I had with a friend, Jack Manning Bancroft. Jack is an Indigenous artist from the Bundjalung nation, who set up AIME (Australian Indigenous Mentoring Experience). 'Creativity is an act of movement, it has purpose,' he tells me. 'We need to think about the circuit of humanity and disrupt the current systems. To move from the networks we have inherited, to the networks we can build, and it's a rainbow, a connection between us all and our imagined states and life beyond the rainbow.'[9]

In *The Body Keeps the Score*, Dr van der Kolk writes that, 'Imagination is absolutely critical to the quality of our lives. Our imagination enables us to leave our routine, everyday existence by fantasizing about travel, food, sex, falling in love, or having the last word – all the things that make life interesting. Imagination gives us the opportunity to envision new possibilities – it is an essential launchpad for making our hopes come true. It fires our creativity, relieves our boredom, alleviates our pain, enhances our pleasure, and enriches our most intimate relationships.'[10]

The prescriptions we share beginning on page 158 of this book are intended to gently open your imagination and make the experience of joy possible by tuning in to glimmers. This is the power of our creativity, but we need to practise it intentionally for this habit to grow and become part of our way of looking at, and experiencing, the world. By looking for glimmers and becoming practised in finding them through creativity, we access a portal to joy, creating a beautiful symbiosis. Through being connected to joy, along with all the other experiences of life, we are closer to our own creativity.

A little note that perhaps joy might need a slight rebrand. It is often portrayed as a state of weightless, fluffy wonder that we just happen to find ourselves in. In reality, we often have to go out and *make* joy, even if it's thin on the ground. We need to jam in the joy whenever we can and, most importantly, when it feels like it's miles away.

> **'Deep down in our minds we have a supercomputer that can set us free: our imagination.'**
>
> **Jack Manning Bancroft**

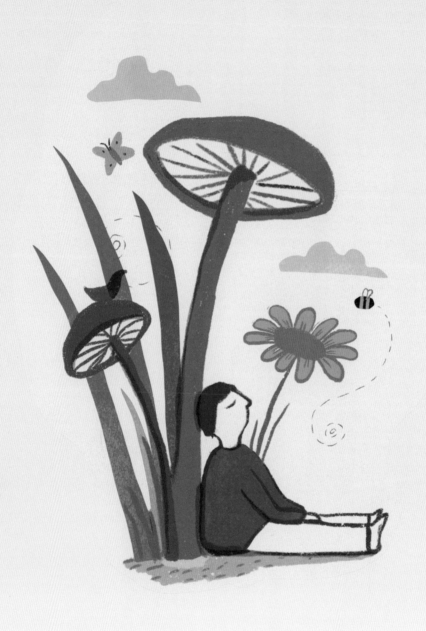

2. Nature

The term 'biophilia' refers to an innate human tendency to connect with nature. It literally translates to 'love of life'.

The symbiotic relationship we share with nature means that we require the benefits of the land, water and air for our survival; we cannot live without it. Not only does nature literally keep us alive, but it can be our medicine, providing tremendous support for our mental health. We evolved deeply immersed in nature, so it's no wonder that being in nature can be a direct support for our brain and nervous system. There are countless studies that show that just sitting in and among trees lowers blood pressure and stress, and boosts mood.[11] The sounds in nature change the connections in our brain and can bring down the fight/flight response, enhancing nervous system function. Being connected to nature, and being connected to creativity, go hand in hand.

In her book *Nature, Our Medicine*, Australian GP Dr Dimity Williams explores the concept of the three-day effect, suggesting that the benefits nature can provide are dose-dependent. Dr Williams cites the work of Dr David Strayer, a cognitive neuroscientist at the University of Utah, who describes how the 'cleaning of the mental windshield' takes three days immersed in the wilderness in order for our busy, exhausted brains to rest and fully recover.[12]

Dr Williams shares a story about how nature assisted her through a very difficult time of grief, following the loss of her mother. 'I had to prioritise nature experiences and commit to them, putting time aside and not allowing other things to get in the way. This has been part of my therapy, like going to a counsellor. I treat it with the same respect, writing a time in my diary and making sure I get there in time to be with myself, in nature.'

Over the years of running our ReMind program, the session with Narelle Happ, a garden designer and horticulturist, remains the one that made the most powerful impact on people, even when we transitioned to Zoom. The simple connection to plants, soil, water – to growing things – seemed to change people in just a few hours.

Field note – Remembering our roots: Andrew's story

Andrew participated in one of our ReMind workshops back in 2020. I caught up with him three years later to check in and see how he was doing and if he'd kept hold of any of the creative practices he'd learnt.

Andrew answers the phone. He sounds like he is digging outside. 'I'm on my way to the greenhouse,' he tells me. I can hear birds chirping and a distant whipper snipper in the background. Andrew takes a breath, apologises for sounding busy and tells me he's been renovating and fixing tiles on the roof wearing thongs, 'because they are the safest footwear'. I question this choice, conjuring an image of Andrew on a roof in iconic Aussie summer sandals. We both laugh.

'I still grapple with what happened to me when I was in the police force every single day, but I'm managing my anxiety now,' he says. Soon we are talking about cacti. He is rattling off lengthy botanical names and speaking of these spiky succulents with fondness, as though they are dear friends.

Andrew tells me he has created a desert in his backyard greenhouse. 'It's sweaty like a steam room – the hybrid varieties love it. I'm with my cactuses every day. I guess tending to all these cacti is kind of mending my mind in some way,' he says.

'At the end of the day, I just look after my collection. It's like therapy. It helps me stay grounded, it brings me joy, and when I have a recurring dream, a regular nightmare, which I often do, well, if I wake up with this dream and go and see my cacti, it calms me down, grounds me again,' he says.

'I had this one cactus while I was working in the cops. It's called old man cactus, *Cephalocereus senilis*, it's really hairy. I was doing general duties shiftwork, so I was pretty tired and busy, and my old man got root bound, I just didn't get around to watering it. Then it just rotted and died. It says a lot, you know, being that disconnected from something that brought me so much joy. It's like forgetting about the old man was a bit like forgetting about myself. I was becoming root-bound too. Finding out about creativity really helped bring me out of my shell. It taught me how to connect again with people safely, and alongside therapy, it really has been such a big part of my healing.'

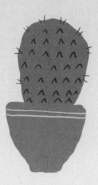

Trees as therapy

One of the most profound face-to-face workshops I have run required no venue booking, materials, catering or data projector. Nature, in all its glory, was the co-facilitator and, to be honest, it was the trees and leaf litter that did most of the work.

On a breezy autumn morning, I took a group of 12 people on a walk through our local rainforest, which is lush with palms, gums, ferns and eucalypts. Trees as Therapy, a two-hour immersive workshop, began with an acknowledgement of the Wodi Wodi people, the traditional owners of that land and forest, followed by a brief grounding practice to bring some calm about being outdoors. The anxiety in the group was visible – discomfort disguised as bravado, or nonchalance.

We shared information about what trees we were looking at, how old they might be and what birds like to live in and around them. We also talked about how trees live in community, their roots pushing through soil underground to connect with each other, to pass nutrients back and forth, to care for each other like a large extended family. At one point we paused at a clearing and I grabbed a book from my bag, *The Hidden Life of Trees*, by German forester Peter Wohlleben. People sat on logs, and in the grass in a circle, and I read aloud a quote that resonated so much more when delivered in the forest with a group of people: 'Trees are like human families: tree parents live together with their children, communicate with them, support them as they grow, share nutrients with those who are sick or struggling, and even warn each other of impending dangers.'[13]

We talked about mycorrhizae – the invisible and vast network of fungi busily at work underground in forests, like a teeny-tiny superhighway of information, nutrients and shared biology connecting roots, soil and insects. We talked about how humans are like that, too; we are designed to reach out and connect with each other. A tree covered with fungi stopped everyone with its wildness for ten whole minutes. Ten out of 12 of the participants cried from joy. Biophilia in action! We walked in silence, with sensory prompts to touch, smell and notice different parts of the forest. Then we gathered in a natural clearing and chatted about the scents of trees and terpenes (compounds that help make the many scents of flowers) and how they emit aromas and natural chemicals that positively impact the human endocrine and immune systems.

We talked about the way that being in a forest locates us in an environment where we are at once both giant and tiny. Right at our feet, almost invisible, are entire colonies and communities of micro insects, whose populations on earth far outnumber us humans, whose world exists mostly in decaying fallen logs from ancient trees – trees that our eyes often see as something hollow or dead, but that are actually teeming with life. We can look up to an enormously tall gum, rock face or boulder, and be reminded just how small we are in the scheme of things, like a speck of dust hurtling through space.

People cried, stopping in their tracks to hug trees. 'It's just been so long, so long, too long, since I've done this,' said one woman who'd been struggling with a range of chronic health issues and was caring for a sick husband.

The impact of this workshop reminded me of a conversation I had with Australian author Charlotte Wood. We talked about connecting with nature as a human right, a political act against capitalism, as a place to disconnect from the market and industry, from advertising. This bunch of people were experiencing what can happen when we do this, and for all of them, me included, it was transformative. Wood also remarked on how almost every writer, artist and creative she knows has a deep practice of nature connection. It is through nature that creative ideas are born.

Nature as medicine

Doctors prescribing a dose of nature to treat mental health issues is on the rise. It seems interesting, though, that given our connection to nature stems so deeply from our evolution, and we literally rely on it for survival, here we are today where nature prescribing in the medical space is seen as an intervention, using terminology such as green treatment and blue treatment, referring to exposure and interaction with grass, parks, hills, and rivers, lakes, the sea.[14] Goodness! Let's remember we are animals – mammals, in fact – and as I already mentioned it is part of our makeup that we must be in nature and, furthermore, that we must play.

I spoke with local GP Dr Mark Melek, who has been working in medical practice for more than 20 years and is an active prescriber of nature and creativity. I wanted to know how this kind of prescribing might look in a clinical setting and, as an example, he shared with me the following excerpt from a recent pair of consultations.

In the first consultation, Patient S told Dr Melek that he was feeling extremely anxious. Dr Melek and Patient S then had a lengthy discussion exploring the basis of these feelings.

Dr Melek then said, 'I would like you to come back in ten days to see if we can figure out a path forward. In the meantime, I'd like you to try something. Please consider this to be an important prescription like any other medication. In fact, I'll even write it down on script paper:

* Swim at least three times, ideally in the ocean, and submerge yourself.
* Go for a walk in the bush once a week, and make sure you feel the bark of the trees with your hands as you go.
* Try a new craft, such as origami. I can also suggest some local workshops that teach ceramics or woodwork.'

Ten days later, Dr Melek asked Patient S how he was feeling. 'I feel like a new man,' Patient S replied. 'I am shocked by this progress and my reduction in anxiety.'

It's important to note here that hiking in the forest or diving into the sea is not possible for many people who live in an urban environment. However, research shows that spending time on a patch of grass or at a local park, or even tending to an indoor plant, can make a difference to your mood.[15] And it's not just plants – wildlife can help us, too. In 2021, German scientists discovered that being in proximity to birdlife offers an increase in life happiness equivalent to $150 a week of added income.[16] Ca-ching! The most important thing is to seek out nature wherever you can. If you can't get yourself out into the wild, it can be helpful to remember that the 'wild' is happening all around us. Nature is fully alive, full of cycles and rhythms that are moving constantly, and tuning in to the rhythm of nature can be effective, too. We can almost always find a way to look up to the sky, make an intention to catch the sunrise or sunset, or catch a cloud passing by.

Dr Melek likened the constant movements and changes in nature to the invisible multi-layered signals that occur within our body every single second. 'There is always something happening,' he tells me. 'We are sent physiological messages almost constantly. When it comes down to it, we all have a sense of innate genius that knows everything about us and how to care for ourselves. Often, it's my job as a GP to allow people a pause, a rest, to enable regulation – a balanced nervous system – so that they can listen to these signals.

'Pathologising feelings and mental illness can take away our agency and may prevent us from asking how or why we are feeling the way we are,' Dr Melek continues. 'We need to support people to catch their breath, to regulate and quieten the "noise" for long enough to be able to listen to this inner wisdom, because it almost certainly knows precisely what we need to do. As practitioners, we need to lean into prescribing modalities that enable pause and connection. It's very hard to listen to your own physiology in a busy world and bustling life, but if we persistently ignore the signals, our mind will eventually take what it needs, even if this means taking us down.

'I'll give you an example,' Dr Melek says, goosebumps already creeping up his arms. 'When I was six I was with my aunty in the car. We drove for what seemed like hours and I remember looking out the window having no idea where I was going, the landscape was so different to the cityscape that I was used to. Eventually we arrived at what I now know as the Police Academy in Goulburn, New South Wales. My aunty's close friend's son was graduating from training, alongside dozens of other officers. My memory from this day is that it was hot, like 40 degrees hot. We were sweating and thirsty and all these police officers were standing dutifully in rows, fully dressed in uniform, blazers, police hats and heavy shoes.

'The sky was blazing blue, not a single cloud in it. I distinctly remember watching these officers standing still and then suddenly they began dropping like flies. It was the first time I'd seen a grown-up collapse. One by one, they fell to the ground, fainting from the heat, the woollen uniforms, the stress. I think about this day quite often and how these people must have been so unattuned with their bodies. They would have been sent countless micro signals of sweating, nausea, light-headedness and perhaps an increased heart rate. Their mind was sending these signals hoping they would take a seat, drink some water, remove their coat or sit in the shade. Eventually if signals are ignored for long enough, and the body senses that its blood supply to the brain is becoming increasingly compromised, the brain takes matters into its own hands. It's as though the mind is speaking to us and eventually says, "Stuff you, I've tried to get your attention. I've tried to take care of us, but you just aren't listening to me. You ignored all my signals. Sorry, but you leave me no choice, I'm going to make you collapse so that we can survive this heat. At least that way I can get the blood flowing back to the brain and we'll be safe." And one by one, they did collapse.'

It made me think of Andrew, who also would have stood there as a new recruit. Spending decades being dictated to by a system of disconnection that trains people to bypass their nervous system responses no doubt contributed to his acute psychological injury, the fallout from which has been devastating. I wonder when and how we became so disconnected?

Ancient wisdom

First Nations Australians have the oldest continuous culture on Earth, living and thriving in deep connection to Country for more than 60,000 years. Indigenous Australians took a creative approach to caring for Country and community using rituals, ceremonies and practices such as song, dance, weaving and storytelling, which have been passed down through generations. As our friend and mentor, Marianne Wobcke, a First Nations midwife, states, 'In Aboriginal culture the relationship between health and wellbeing and connection to Country is paramount. It is therefore essential that the foundation of any health initiatives embraces this understanding of the importance of Country in a spiritual, physical, intellectual, social and cultural context.'[17] We have so much to learn from First Nations Australians' knowledge systems in terms of care, how they look after themselves, each other and the environment.

Living and learning from nature is part of our history, and the more I work with people who are experiencing symptoms of mental ill health, the more I recognise the necessity of remembering this way of life as a vital remedy. As Aboriginal scholar Tyson Yunkaporta says, 'All humans evolved within complex, land-based cultures over deep time to develop a brain with the capacity for over 100 trillion neural connections, of which we now only use a tiny fraction. Most of us have been displaced from those cultures of origin, a global diaspora of refugees severed not only from land, but from the sheer genius that comes from belonging in symbiotic relation to it.'[18]

Recognising and applying a practice of creativity to manage health is slowly making its way into policy discussions. Creative Australia (formerly Australia Council for the Arts) recently released a report stating that creativity can extend beyond traditional health services to address the social determinants of health. This is due to the power of creative experiences to facilitate engagement with, and connections for, people with diverse lived experience.[19]

Through our work at MakeShift – working with people like Kate and Andrew, and discussing nature prescribing with Dr Melek – Caitlin and I decided to learn how to bring the wisdom of First Nations culture into the setting of creative prescribing. In 2022, I participated in a customised program, My Place on Country, run by change maker and Yuin woman Linda Kennedy, from Future Black.

My place on Country

'Where are you from?' This question was posed to a group of MakeShift staff, board members and creative facilitators during My Place on Country, a four-week course designed to develop skills and abilities in cross-cultural engagement. The program aims to empower participants to engage with their own relationship to Country, and to deeply understand the impacts of colonisation. We participated in this program in the thick of the pandemic, when living in the unknown and unfamiliar became everyone's reality. In a small way, coming together to learn about connection and forming a relationship to Dharawal Country, the land upon which we all lived, felt like sending down roots, and helped to keep us all grounded, in place and safe.

'Who are your ancestors?' Linda asked us. I was stumped. I knew where I was born, where my folks were born, but my knowledge beyond that was limited. What about my grandparents and their mothers and fathers? I felt untethered and a tiny bit hollow, so I began digging through my family history, unearthing documents and gathering stories, until I was able to piece together parts of my heritage. I learnt the name of the land on which I was born, I discovered how and why my parents first came to Australia. Pulling together small pieces of knowledge where I could helped create a sense of belonging, and I began to orient myself to my local environment.

My Place on Country created a profound sense of togetherness within the group and gave us all permission to connect with Country in a way we hadn't previously. Walking on our local land soon became a curious exercise in finding and sharing. We were like a bunch of excited schoolkids swapping tales about the moonrise or a lyrebird sighting or stumbling upon a vibrant thread of jewel bugs. Curiosity was contagious and it helped to grow our creativity. We had all become veritable glimmer hunters. From the depths of this program, poems were written, paintings created, photos taken and a giant collection of stories harvested to pass on.

'All humans evolved
within complex,
land-based cultures
over deep time to develop
a brain with the capacity
for over 100 trillion
neural connections, of
which we now only use
a tiny fraction.'

———

Tyson Yunkaporta

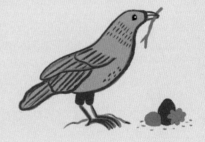

3. Community

Just as trees depend upon each other, helping neighbours in times of need,[20] so do humans. Humans are designed to live in groups. We are social creatures who require meaningful connections. In today's society it can be harder to cultivate community in the way that it shaped us thousands of years ago. The act of creativity is a powerful way to sustain connections between people and to ultimately foster a sense of community. We talk about this in more detail in Chapter 4, when we explore the nervous system. We will show you how our biology is actually imprinted and hardwired to reach out and find connections with others, and that primal impulse never, ever leaves us.

Let's meet Vince. It was when Vince turned up on Zoom towards the end of a ReMind program with a hand-stitched lorikeet that I knew something was working. Vince was in the police force for 23 years. I met him when he'd swapped his uniform for Hawaiian shirts. He was really struggling with PTSD and had tried a plethora of therapies. We chatted about surfing and things that made him feel good: his mum, sunsets, cars and anything that lifted the weight of angst that he was feeling after being medically retired from the force. 'I'm not creative,' he told me, 'but I'll try anything.' That was all I needed to hear and we were off and away.

It wasn't easy for Vince to ring the doorbell on the Zoom room, but he did for eight weeks, and over that time he went from not getting out of bed in the morning to cooking his family dinner from scratch most nights and calling his mum every Sunday to do embroidery together.

Vince told me he would put the phone on loud speaker so his hands could keep stitching. His mum, Norma, started embroidery when she learnt from her mother at age ten. She mended and stitched her whole life. Vince had never threaded a needle.

After one session with textile artist Michele Elliot and me on Zoom, Vince went from making lines with thread to hand-stitching lorikeets. He went on to do this every Sunday with his mum, over the phone, until he had a menagerie! Keeping his hands busy kept his brain calm; stitching with his mum was easier than finding things to talk about. Slowly he was connecting with himself, with her and with the world, and this unexpected practice of stitching became a trusty companion he could depend upon.

Vince later told me that embroidering was not something that he could have imagined doing 'in a million years'. But through this experience, Vince began to connect with both his family and the larger community, specifically the ReMind participants.

Like Vince's threads, stories carry us through our days. We are incessantly creating them and they can really assist us to make meaning of life, as well as filling us up with feel-good hormones. When we deeply listen to stories, it changes our brain chemistry, flooding it with oxytocin, which builds empathy. This exchange is the core of building trust and connection.

Our work at MakeShift has been driven by a deep urge to find ways for people to connect through shared interests, passions and ideas instead of shared problems. Finding glimmers of joy, like Vince stitching lorikeets or Kate noticing stars, produces feel-good hormones in the person experiencing the moment of joy. There's also a wonderful after-effect: we almost always want to share what we have experienced when it comes from a pleasurable state. Passing on glimmers becomes irresistible!

Storytelling

Humans have been practising a deep connection to creativity and sharing stories in some form or another for tens of thousands of years. These stories first began as visual representations (cave drawings, hieroglyphs, etc.) and from there an oral tradition developed, which remains one of the strongest and most common creative acts we all do today. All of us are storytellers. As Deb Dana, who coined the term glimmers, says, 'We humans are storytellers, meaning-making beings, and it is through our autonomic nervous systems that we first create, and then inhabit, our stories.'[21]

The act of creativity offers a way to write and rewrite the stories we tell about ourselves. We know that the most fundamental experiences humans require are to be seen and to belong. Finding joy, connecting to nature and being in community are reliable ways of helping us reach this state of belonging. This is not an easy feeling to cultivate. It doesn't happen overnight – it takes practice and effort – but by virtue of design we do have the tools we need inside us to ultimately look after ourselves and each other. Agency is important, and storytelling – 'telling our stories' – can be the framework that enables us to experience belonging.

Agency is right at the heart of creative first aid. It's about applying creativity as a requirement for mending. We must tend to ourselves daily in order to mend, and as human beings with a nervous system, this cycle of tending and mending is almost constant, much like the constant cycles of nature.

At a nature connection retreat in 2022, Caitlin and I listened to Andrew Turbill (aka The Bird Guy) talk about observing birds and wildlife, and how adult humans do this nifty thing where our brain invents the story of what we think is there, to save time, instead of really looking at what is actually there. So we might see a woman riding down the street on a bicycle and imperceptibly our brain has already invented the story of her slowing down for the traffic light, nanoseconds before she actually has. He stressed the importance of really looking, with eyes and ears, to make sure we take in the detail of what we see, not just what we think we see. This reflects the power of storytelling in our circuitry – that it is truly hardwired in our nature to invent, to create, to make.

I spoke with storyteller and author Dr Paul Callaghan, a First Nations Worimi man, about storytelling. It didn't take long for our conversation to become an act of sharing tales about ourselves. One of his biggest stories was about how connecting to Country saved his life. 'Depression has been my greatest teacher. It's what got me back on Country, which is the very reason I am still here today, literally. Country is where you connect in mind and spirit. It's about relationship with place and everything, including animals, rocks, plants and people. In our tradition, everything has a story.'

In 2022, Dr Callaghan and Uncle Paul Gordon published *The Dreaming Path*. In their book, they write that 'When we leave this world, we leave behind our stories. Everything is connected to story and art is the means that enables us to go beyond head and to feel. It's not just about heart, it's about our gut feeling, our inner wisdom.'[22]

'Creativity and the arts enable us to become our authentic selves as truth tellers,' Dr Callaghan explained to me. 'The arts can't be fudged like fact and figures, and I'm highly trained in commerce, so I know! It allows us to be authentic and to find and shape our story. We all have a story.' Art provides a menu of transferring data into intuitive wisdom. A creative act that comes from this place of intuitive wisdom dissolves all the critical voices – the imposter, the judge, the shaming voice. When you tune in to your innate creativity and explore it, not for the reader, or an audience, but for the spirits and for Country, then it's in that connection that deep mindfulness happens. It can be incredibly healing.

'When you have a story, you also have a song, and when you have a song, you also have a dance. Story is our way of communicating and sharing knowledge. We can't ever stop telling and listening to stories. It's integral to being human!' These words from Dr Callaghan played out in real life when our work at MakeShift took me into the juvenile justice setting.

Stories through song

The kids in Reiby Juvenile Justice Centre are separated by gender. Boys in green T-shirts and black shorts, girls in maroon tops and black trackpants. The staff hold giant bunches of keys and wear small earpiece microphones at all times. Each week, I go to Reiby with an artist to bring creativity to the young people on the inside, as a form of creative first aid. The room we work from is full of chairs called mental health furniture. Kids can sit in deep cone-shaped pods that have weighted arm blankets to wrap around themselves. These chairs end up co-facilitating with us, keeping the kids safe and grounded while they absorb the content we're delivering.

This week, the artist joining me is Nooky, a First Nations hip-hop artist and proud Yuin and Thungutti man known for his no-holds-barred, hyperactive brand of rap. He keeps words and direction to a minimum, instead letting the music run the session. Nooky connects through kinship, nodding, 'Hi sis', 'Hi bro', while he sets up his gear. Loud music greets the kids as they arrive. Rap music, quick beats – they seem to know exactly what to do as they enter the room, nodding or high-fiving Nooky and then settling in.

I've put a pen and paper out for each kid and within ten minutes they've all got lyrics written down. The hectic backbeats are on a constant loop, while the kids mouth silent rhymes to themselves, rapidly scribbling down words and nodding their heads rhythmically. Nooky and the music do all the subtle crafting of this session, until I get passed sheets of paper by one of the girls. 'Do you reckon this works, sis?' I'm asked. We spend a chunk of time together, swapping words, shaping rhymes. The kids' lyrics are pulled straight from their hearts; they're telling stories through rap that they otherwise couldn't.

One girl writes a chorus, wedged between a bunch of super-fast beats. 'Can you sing this bit, the chorus, and rap the verse?' I ask. She grabs the microphone and lays down her freestyle rap about being stuck in a cell, in a system, about wanting to say sorry to her family, about wanting to go home. Her chorus brings the room to complete silence. The kids, the staff, Nooky, we're all suspended momentarily by her singing. Her voice, like a shooting star, arrived from nowhere. I catch tears falling down my face.

The young people in juvenile justice are some of the state's most vulnerable, many of them born into trauma. Using creativity to forge tiny pathways of connection is their human right. We all deserve to experience moments of joy, or nature, or community, no matter what our story is.

Weaving the threads

At the heart of all the stories I've shared here is this: the role of joy, nature and community is deeply woven into the history and lifetime of human experience. We have always been seekers of these things. But in the past few hundred years, how we organise, work and inhabit places has changed so dramatically that we've gradually moved away from experiencing connection to these fundamental human needs.

It requires an intentional desire to find even the threads of these three vital parts of being human. Community can be elusive in busy, urban neighbourhoods, as can nature. Joy is hard to find when basic needs like housing, work and health care are under threat. Practising creative first aid gives us a little path towards these things. They are there, and always have been. They are sometimes obscured. We might need some binoculars and some good hiking boots, but this adventure is absolutely worth taking.

✳ **Field note** – Tending imperfect gardens: Janice's story

Janice was a paramedic for 12 years, working in the fast-paced streets of Sydney before serving in regional New South Wales. She'd reached the point in her career she had hoped for, to become a clinical training manager. When she joined MakeShift's ReMind program, she was only recently out of hospital, and, in her words, acutely unwell. Her PTSD symptoms and depression were severe, and it was an incredibly fragile and frightening time in her life. 'Being hospitalised saved my life. But having had one foot in the biomedical model as a paramedic and one foot as a patient suffering from PTSD, meant I really got to see both sides. I realised that there's not one thing that fixes us. There's not one pill, not one intervention. We are all so different and it's about figuring out what we need. I really strongly believe we are our own best therapists. Well that's been my experience, anyway.' Janice shared her story with us.

'I worked in a job that demanded perfection, but it was unreasonable to have complete perfection in an emergency situation. Every day I was striving to respond perfectly, to do the best I could, always and relentlessly. I was in a loop of being on high alert and trying hard to keep everything controlled. In ReMind, being given permission to just

mess around and play, to make mistakes and make something just for the sake of making, well I realised years later that this was a really powerful intervention. It was medicinal for me and is what has had the biggest impact on me in my healing.

'I go to this space of mess and imperfection now all the time in my garden. Before I used to think I had to create a perfect garden, but in fact gardens change all the time. ReMind taught me to enjoy the constant changes of my plants and the soil. I no longer strive to have a perfect garden, I just love being grounded in the earth, with my two loyal doggos close by.

'Nobody knows us as well as we know ourselves, and that's why I think creativity and creative practice played an enormous role in my recovery. I got to practise this feeling by being creative, a tiny bit at a time, little by little, with drawing, gardening, writing, and over time I guess I was able to apply this to myself in my life, to fully let go of things that I couldn't control.

'What I have learnt is that creativity, exercise, self-care, a lot of therapy and good support have been essential ingredients for me to stay well. Oh, and also my dog!'

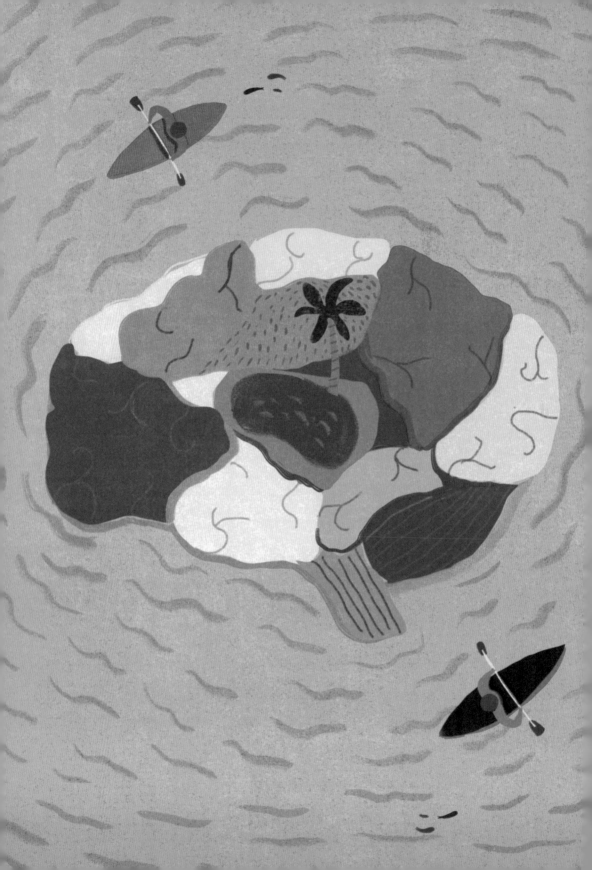

CHAPTER 4

Brain Wave:
Saying hello to your
nervous system

by Caitlin

In the midst of the Covid lockdowns of 2020, our family adopted a pandemic puppy (I know, what a cliché) – a sensitive, open-hearted, on-the-job border collie we named Bowie. His vigilance in keeping us all safe – following our every move, barking at every innocuous person walking calmly down our street, even sitting in the corner of the bathroom while I shower – is a lot. It's his primal instinct to protect in this way, but the training has had to be consistent and intentional to balance that instinct with a calm, happy household.

Bowie is a bit like our nervous system, which we are going to explore in this chapter. Its purpose is to constantly and vigilantly read thousands of imperceptible cues of potential danger, and react with our own safety as its number one priority. Learning to 'read' our nervous system responses can help us manage our mental wellbeing, and these responses can be adjusted, as for Bowie, through consistent practice and awareness.

The way we experience the world through emotions, thoughts and behaviours is triaged and managed by an internal ground control known as the autonomic nervous system (ANS). (I always found this term amusing, with a vague memory of high school biology conjuring up images of a machine-like sea creature full of jangly nerves – wide-eyed, anxious and scared.) To keep things clean and simple here, we will refer to it simply as the nervous system.

The nervous system is a complex and sophisticated living network made up of the brain, spinal cord and a web of nerves that traverse most of the body. It also includes the largest nerve in the body, the vagus nerve, which starts at the stem of the brain and travels all the way to the base of the spine and abdomen. As a whole, the nervous system, which has two main components – the sympathetic and the parasympathetic – helps different parts of the body communicate, and controls the automatic responses we have, including breathing, swallowing, walking, learning. It is also the central hub for our reactions, coordinating our responses to danger, stress, threat and distress.

The nervous system is like the conductor of an orchestra with three sections, working to keep it in balance.

Rest and digest is the state where connection is possible, and there is a felt sense of safety and security. The nervous system has decided we are not under threat, and can relax and let the other parts of our brain sit up front, taking the wheel so that we can connect with others, feel compassion, learn new information, and use logic and creativity. It can also be referred to as the **ventral vagal state.**

Freeze and collapse is almost the opposite of fight and flight. The automatic survival-mechanism trigger senses that safety is best reached by being totally numbed, frozen, still or a complete pushover. This is sometimes referred to as the **dorsal vagal state**, dorsal meaning 'back' – the back branch of the vagus nerve. This branch responds to cues of danger by moving into numb, frozen shutdown.

Fight and flight is the responsive state that occurs when the **sympathetic** nervous system is triggered by perceived danger or threat. It's often an automatic reaction that we're not aware of until it is happening, but it's a core survival trait of mammals. In this state the possibility of connection, open-ness and compassion is closed off, survival being the number one priority.

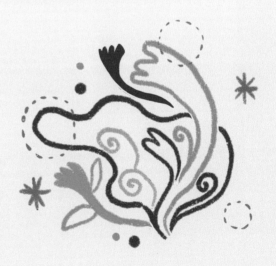

The keys to our wellbeing

When it comes to how we feel and perceive our sense of safety, the nervous system is always on the job, scanning and interpreting hundreds of almost imperceptible cues from our own body and the external world, making assessments in microseconds as to the degree of danger we face. Its priority is twofold: survival and staying safe, and connection.

We'll explore the fight/flight, rest/digest and freeze/collapse states in more detail later in this chapter. It's probably a good moment to mention that it's difficult to do a proper job of this without referring to a bunch of technical terms. You don't need to get too hung up on them, but knowing about the different vagal states is worthwhile. It's useful to build your knowledge of these terms, particularly as the origins of them stem from 'polyvagal theory', a relatively recent and exciting new paradigm for understanding human emotions, behaviour, psychology and trauma. (There are some suggestions of further reading on page 257 if you'd like more detail on polyvagal theory, which underpins this content about the nervous system.)

When it comes to understanding the term 'ventral vagal state', I think about it as the double 'V' sign – peace out! In this state, everything is pretty great, chill and cruisy. It's our window for the ideal conditions for our life.

There is a tendency to think of mental health as being simply about the mind, e.g. our brain delivering unhelpful and discordant thought patterns that disrupt our capacity to feel and act in healthy ways. But in fact, our mental wellbeing depends on the state of both our mind *and* body. We say 'mind and body' almost unthinkingly, but an important part of this particular wander through our internal circuitry is understanding that our minds are part of our bodies. They are not separate entities, but part of an elegant ecosystem all working together and harmonising in mostly invisible ways.

We referred to the concept of regulation earlier. Regulation is our ability to harness some control of our emotional responses to our experiences. To be dysregulated is to be very far away from that 'rest and digest' state, which means being quite disconnected from reason, rational thinking, logic and nuance.

While much of the way our nervous system works is automatic and occurs outside of the logical, thinking brain, it is completely possible to learn mindful strategies to notice some of the signs of dysregulation. From there we can apply a range of practices that are very effective in bringing the nervous system back into balance. Beginning to understand our nervous system and how we can manage it is vital to being able to live in ways that maximise our psychological wellbeing, no matter what life throws at us.

You probably weren't taught in school how to regulate your nervous system. So it's not surprising that when we experience anxiety and depression and burnout, we are encouraged to head straight to the doctor instead of tuning in to our nervous system.

Becoming mates with our nervous system empowers us to reach a state where we can make good decisions about what it will take to live well, feel well and even thrive. This comes with recognising the responses of our nervous system, and being able to apply strategies that work to bring this system into balance. Strategies like cold-water swimming, creative writing, dancing in your lounge room, walking in nature, mark-making, singing and making craft all do this job really effectively. How cool is that?

Let's wave hello

So let's come back to the basics. We are human. We are limited by the design of the human body, which is extraordinary and can withstand an incredible amount. We need food, water and shelter to survive, for our bodies not to wither and die.

But in order to bring meaning to our lives, we need other things, too. We need purpose and connection and the space and opportunity to mend after great challenges. And we need regular moments of rest and replenishment for our minds and bodies to keep going.

We are not built to work without breaks and function at high speed without resetting our nervous system. We are not designed to withstand months, even years, of stress. Tricia Hersey, US artist, author of *Rest is Resistance*, and founder of The Nap Ministry,[1] an organisation that 'examines the liberating power of naps', explains that when we are totally exhausted, being able to be creative is impossible, our intuition and capacity to imagine being so limited by a society that promotes overworking.

If we were to set out for a day-long walk across a hot, dry landscape, we would plan for it accordingly. We would put on hiking boots, fill a water bottle and wear a wide-brimmed hat. We accept this, and don't question it.

Yet, bewilderingly, we question our own capability when we are depleted, despairing and anxious because we haven't given our psychological systems what they need to thrive, or even survive. We label ourselves as unproductive or broken when we struggle to cope in circumstances that don't allow us to replenish and rest our nervous system.

That's not some personal flaw of millions of people. We are getting those messages from the culture we live in. The lines between work and home are pretty darn blurry when our office can be housed in the smartphone in our pocket. That particular amazing technology, along with 24-hour news cycles and social media, has created an environment of constant alert, alarm, news and tsunami-level waves of information coming at us, all day every day. To adjust to that reality, we need to make tending to our nervous system a priority.

We all have mental health, that being the status of our psychological functioning, and it shifts and changes according to life and all the things in it. For some people, the absence of major hardships and the presence of things like a supportive, close family and community, and financial security, can result in pretty stable, unwavering mental health status. Active practices of self-care can help maintain this status.

In talking about those who live with mental health challenges, we refer primarily to experiences that come with labels like depression, anxiety and trauma, but of course, many people live with highly complex diagnoses of psychiatric illnesses. Applying creative first aid is useful for everyone, but we acknowledge that these situations call for a considered, individualised medical treatment journey.

There is also a significant rise in the diagnosis of conditions like ADHD and autism. The day to day of living with this reality means that some of the ways neurodivergence occurs for people are put in the same basket as 'mental health issues', when they are in fact different experiences.

This spectrum shouldn't be pathologised. The social model of disability[2] says that people are disabled by the attitudes and structures of society, and so we don't need to 'fix' people and their 'symptoms', but rather shift and change our culture to include, accommodate and also celebrate these diverse experiences of the world. That is also a lens we bring to this conversation, and we tend to refer to symptoms as 'experiences', mostly for this reason.

It is undeniable that throughout each of our lives, we will all experience impacts to our mental wellbeing, to some degree, and being prepared for this reality is the best chance we have at protecting our mental health. We can do this by befriending, responding to and healing our nervous system.

This is something we can begin immediately, one minute at a time, making tiny steps towards being grounded and present and in a regulated space to keep making good decisions. To cultivate the tiny moments where that inner voice might get to call out to us, and we can truly listen to what it tells us. It is a true act of body knowledge, self-compassion and creativity. A great place to start this personal investigative process is learning about the Window of Tolerance.

The Window of Tolerance

The Window of Tolerance is a great tool to use when we begin this journey through the nervous system. Developed by clinical psychiatrist Dr Dan Siegel, the Window of Tolerance[3] is our ideal, optimal state of functioning, where we can sail smoothly through our days, meeting stress and responsibility with resilience and rational thinking.

Our window is widened when we experience connection, safety and mindfulness. But that same window can be narrowed by experiences of persistent stress, trauma, danger and isolation.

The Window of Tolerance refers to the state where our nervous system is in balance. The 'rest/digest' state, and the 'fight/flight' state, specifically, are in harmony. The latter state is, and has always been, essential for the survival of the human race.[4] It is a mobilising state of motivation and action and, like most things, is a spectrum that shifts and changes.

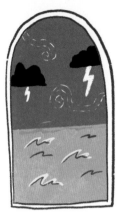
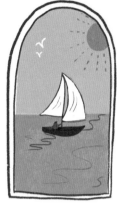
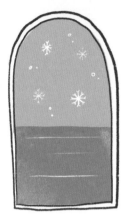

Fight/Flight
Emotional overwhelm, panic; feeling unsafe, angry, wired, anxious

Rest/Digest (ventral vagal)
Carrying on with daily life in our Window of Tolerance

Freeze/Collapse
Numb, disconnected, dissociated, no energy, exhausted, withdrawn, shut down

Just as we suggest for practising creativity, a little inch-by-inch thinking is useful here in refraining from seeing any of these nervous system states as 'good' or 'bad'. All of them are necessary and have a role to play. What's positive or healthy for our wellbeing is having some agency in controlling how much our nervous system swings between these states, and some capacity to influence it.

Being in your Window of Tolerance doesn't mean everything is just bloody lovely. But it does mean that you are in a state where you are able to:

✳ learn new information
✳ solve problems
✳ show compassion for others
✳ be creative and innovative
✳ meet stress with resilience and action
✳ feel safe
✳ remain mindful and open.

Each person's Window of Tolerance is unique and depends on multiple factors. Rest assured that having a narrow window or regularly being outside your Window of Tolerance when you go through challenging and terrible experiences is completely normal. This is simply an unconscious need to survive and protect yourself. Understanding this also can help us foster more self-compassion, as we realise that experiencing an absence of compassion, or being quick to anger, isn't happening because we are awful, terrible people. These are normal responses to being outside our Window of Tolerance.

Furthermore, we can actually train our nervous system to slowly widen that window, inch by inch. And one of the best ways to do this is through intentional creative practices. In fact, we share 50 of them later in this book, starting on page 158. Our brains are plastic, after all! It's why even short, micro practices that cue our nervous system to reset and relax help us return to that Window of Tolerance. Over time, these practices create well-trodden paths in our brain's neural superhighway, making the activities easier to return to again and again.

Returning home

Vagus means 'wander' in Latin. Deb Dana, a clinician and consultant who specialises in complex trauma, describes being in our Window of Tolerance (the ventral vagal state) as being 'home'.[5] And moving from that state into dysregulation can be thought of as wandering away from home.

Learning to be comfortable and familiar in this 'home' (rest and digest) state might best be achieved by thinking about these kinds of questions:

✳ What does it feel like to be home (home being a place of safety and comfort)?
✳ What are the things we miss when we are away from home?
✳ What are the furnishings we need to make home a safe haven for our souls?

We could say that we wander far from home, or are outside our Window of Tolerance, when our nervous system moves in one of two directions: flight/flight or freeze/collapse. We can think about travelling away from the home of our comfort window when we are activated in a dysregulated state. Of course, leaving home is unavoidable, and required at certain times, but what's important is that we know how to return. Before we do that, let's learn more about these two states: fight or flight; and freeze or collapse.

Fight or flight

Characterised by feelings of panic, dread, fear and anger, the fight-or-flight state is common to everyone, but for some of us it's the default setting. Often called 'hyper-arousal', this physiological reaction occurs in response to a perceived threat and causes intense energy to flood our system with adrenaline and cortisol. It is an essential survival mechanism that would have enabled us to outrun wild animals or these days even lift a car off a pram with a baby trapped inside.

The supermarkets of March 2020 were full of folks in this state. Anger, aggression and buying all the toilet paper was bewildering to behold, but when we zoom out and think about it, it makes a lot of sense. The perceived global threat certainly was real enough to trigger this response of humans to gather resources, stay alert, defend and control territory as a means of ensuring safety. It also brought a real, active traumatic sense that we were in danger and couldn't see loved ones, and that many people were going to (and did) die. It's no wonder the numbers of those feeling anxious, exhausted and overwhelmed are so high.

Symptoms of the fight-or-flight state are wide-ranging. They can be physical, such as:

* heart palpitations
* sweaty palms
* shaky hands
* churning stomach
* heavy chest
* pounding head
* wobbly legs
* racing thoughts
* inability to focus.

They can also be emotional, leaving us feeling:

✳ hypervigilant, as if danger is lurking around the corner
✳ a sense of panic, dread and fear
✳ wired, awake, full of adrenaline
✳ overwhelmed, irritated and angry
✳ disconnected from our heart, and far away from compassion and empathy. By golly, that's because our nervous system DOESN'T HAVE TIME! It's busy keeping us safe from imminent danger.

In this state, we might try to project-manage our life, barging through sensitive moments like a dog charging through a picnic. It means we will likely miss nuanced cues and information that in fact the world isn't against us, and that people are actually trying to help. This can lead to intense feelings of mistrust, fear, defensiveness and aggressive energy.

We are not designed to remain, week in and week out, in this hypervigilant state, so we crash, giving way to the most primal, most ancient system of human design – freeze or collapse, or hypo-arousal.

Practices to inch away from fight-or-flight states

Certain practices can be helpful in shifting our nervous system out of the fight-or-flight state. These activities tend to be sensory, somatic and sometimes quite physical, such as:

✳ engaging in cardio exercise
✳ swimming or taking showers in cold water
✳ listening to loud, rhythmic music
✳ dancing or shaking[6]
✳ gardening – heavy lifting, weeding, mulching, etc.
✳ painting, drawing
✳ making things – knitting, using clay, weaving, sewing, building Lego, etc.
✳ cooking.

Each of these activities requires repetitive actions that help us to regulate our nervous system and slow down that hyper-aroused, frenetic energy coursing through us.

It can feel counterintuitive that to offset heightened, frenzied experiences we don't necessarily need to engage in calm, gentle activities. Often it can be best to meet this with an equal intensity of vigorous sensory input. While short and impactful practices can make an immediate difference, the effect is even greater when we turn them into habits, well-worn paths that our brain finds familiar and understands as a cue to relax.

My busy head tends to lean towards this activated, mobilised state at the first hint of stress or threat, and the heavy sense of dread in my chest is the first sign, often arriving when I least expect it. I've come to learn that a quick jump in the water, no matter the time of year, is like an incredible reset button for my entire sense of feeling. Loud, heavy music through headphones also calms these sensations, along with some intense exercise such as lifting heavy things, or dancing.

Freeze or collapse

This response system works to de-escalate or escape threat and danger through stillness, or compliance. Much like the fight-or-flight state, this protective response kicks into gear when we are faced with incredible pain or stress. However, in this state the nervous system's best perceived response to threat is to curl up, be small, stay still and play dead. It can manifest as complete and utter bone-tired exhaustion, a fatigue so powerful it shuts down all other functions. Or as fawning, when we go along with whatever someone else wants as a strategy to placate them, and remove the possibility of displeasure, anger or danger being directed at us.

For years after my mother died, on her birthday I would wake up full of reasonable, sensible intentions to mark the day in some way: perhaps a visit to the botanic gardens or playing her favourite music. Instead, I would often find myself overcome with the most unusual, heady fatigue, like I'd been drugged, and then I'd sleep for hours in the middle of the day. This was not a conscious or logical process in my brain. More recently, when I found myself suddenly and surprisingly opening boxes of my mother's things - diaries, letters, journals from her time of illness, I had the same, almost instant response of complete shutdown and exhaustion, unable to take decisive action.

'The ability to respond to and recover from the challenges of daily living is a marker of wellbeing and depends on the actions of the autonomic nervous system.'

—

Deb Dana

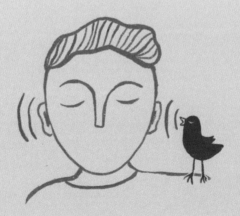

Hypo-arousal can also come in the form of total numbness. Disassociating is a powerful protective mechanism of the nervous system, and when the threat or pain is just too much to bear, our clever brain shields us by feeling absolutely nothing at all.

Other symptoms of the freeze-and-collapse state include:

* foggy headedness
* feelings of despair and hopelessness
* lack of energy and pleasure in life
* a loss of motivation
* heavy or floppy limbs.

Like the fight/flight state, our nervous system is prioritising survival instead of connection. To be in this freeze/collapse state for extended periods can numb us to all of life's experiences – the painful, but also the joyful, delightful moments. It can make disconnection and a sense of pointlessness feel normal and familiar. As trauma research pioneer Dr Bessel van der Kolk says, 'You cannot do psychotherapy or psychoeducation when people are frozen, because when you're frozen, nothing can come into your brain until the frozenness is stopped.'[7]

Practices to inch away from freeze-or-collapse states

If we think about the activities for disrupting the fight-or-flight state as vigorous, sensory practices that meet the level of energy we're already experiencing, then for this state the practices should be a lot less intense.

Research shows[8] that gentle and still sensory experiences like the ones listed below can provide the most relief:

* engaging your sense of smell (i.e. smelling flowers, food, etc.)
* looking at nature
* reading poetry
* slow stretching
* listening to relaxing music
* gentle movement or dancing

* creative writing or doodling
* easy, gentle drawing, crafting or knitting.

Again, many of these practices can act as a kind of repetitive meditation, helping us find that state of flow and return to our Window of Tolerance. Sometimes it might be simple humming, or slow movement and stretching that kickstarts this process.

Where am I? Have I wandered far from home?

It can be helpful to regularly ask ourselves this question, helping us stay connected to mindful awareness of our nervous system state. Instead of jumping to the conclusion that we are broken or unwell if we feel dread or anxiety, connecting with our nervous system helps us learn that this is simply a moment in time, and it too shall pass.

These days, it is not uncommon for the average person to live with an unsustainable level of stress. From our cultural obsession with work and the ever-increasing cost of living, to the lack of community support and constant barrage of social media right at our fingertips, the list of ingredients in this society-wide stress soup is long. It is not surprising that remaining in our Window of Tolerance has become harder and harder.

So how do we change that? Firstly, by taking a moment of reflection each day to collect data on where we are in relation to our Window of Tolerance.

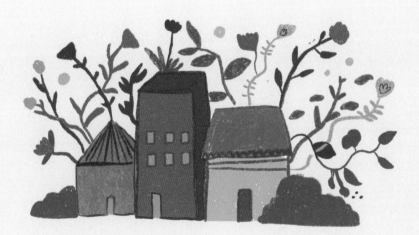

Start by listening
to your body

If even beginning to notice where you are in terms of your Window of Tolerance seems tricky (which it is for some, as living with trauma can mean being very disconnected from knowing how you feel), you could start with a simple body scan exercise. Body scan is the mindful process of checking in, from head to toe and fingertip to toe, and noticing any sensations, tension or signals. It is a great practice for building the skill of tuning in to all the messages our body is sending.

This exercise helps us tune in to the messages, both loud and also almost imperceptible, that our body is giving us. Our body actually tells us things all the time. Many of us are trained, even as children, to ignore these messages: to soldier on when we are sick, or to ignore that gut feeling when someone sets off alarm bells when we're in their presence.

In the same way that we don't have to remember to blink, our stress response systems draw upon a multitude of micro cues within the body to determine their response. This is known as neuroception. Our internal surveillance system is designed to be constantly absorbing information from our body and using that to determine how to respond, with survival and safety the evergreen and sole priority.

There are many functions of the human body like this. We all breathe without thinking about it, even while sleeping. And we know that there are techniques we can intentionally use to improve the quality of our breathing, to bring some mindfulness to it, and enrich and maximise how much oxygen we bring into our lungs. We can apply the same process to meeting and getting to know our nervous system. While we'll never be able to fully hear and see this invisible process, we can learn to pay a little more attention to it.

Interoception, by contrast, is the sensations we have of our internal organs and body mechanics, like feeling thirsty, hungry or sweaty, even sensing our own heartbeat. By mindfully noticing these things, we can slowly start tuning in to those more invisible, unconscious experiences.

Another practice that can really bring us closer to these sensations is called elements meditation.

Begin by asking yourself the following questions:

✳ **Earth:** Do I feel heaviness or lightness anywhere in my body (e.g. heavy feet, light head)?
✳ **Air:** Is there movement or stillness somewhere in my body (e.g. fluttery heart, numb legs)?
✳ **Fire:** Do I have sensations of hotness or coldness in my body (e.g. cold hands, sweaty, hot head)?
✳ **Water:** Can I sense dryness or moisture in my body, inside or out (e.g. dry face, watery eyes)?

The first step in using the Window of Tolerance lens is to begin to take note of the little messages our body already clearly sends us, such as body temperature, hunger, heartbeat. We are rewiring ourselves to take these messages seriously. Our bodies know what they need, so these two activities: body scan and elements meditation, can help us start building this skill.

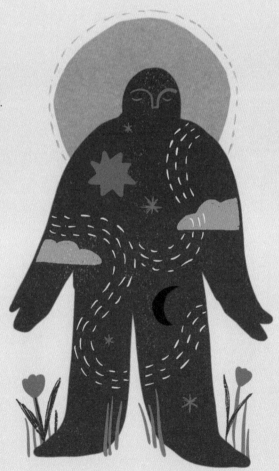

How to keep returning home

In applying the lens of the Window of Tolerance, we can try to begin taking notice of how our nervous system is primed to respond. This is a little harder and requires some practice at tuning in to body knowledge. If we were curious about what we noticed over a week, or two, would there be a pattern? The mindful noticing of such patterns is just that – mindful. We don't need to judge or think of any moments and days we are outside this window of regulation as 'bad' or some kind of failure. It is a message from our body asking us to do something.

Being propelled out of a regulated state can creep up on us. It can actually accumulate inch by inch, from a little irritability here, some overreactions there, to suddenly feeling that all-encompassing dread, panic, overwhelm and physical discomfort. If you've been fortunate enough to have a relatively grief- and trauma-free life so far, your nervous system may be superbly in balance, and not set on a default to over-respond even to small things. It's still useful to support your nervous system, kind of like a raincoat in heavy rain – just because you're okay with the rain, you don't always want to get wet!

It's taken me a while to learn, notice and reflect back later to recognise the early signs that I'm wandering away from my rest-and-digest state. The all too predictable catastrophising: 'Oh, surely my partner is late because there's been a terrible train crash.' The little twitch of unsettled dread; the snapping at my kids; a heavy, pressing sensation in my chest; and then quickly abandoning good habits – these are all the cues that I'm heading out the door and into a dysregulated place of fight or flight.

In the same way that wandering away from our Window of Tolerance (our optimal state of being) can be a slow or incredibly swift (but most often imperceptible) process, returning home can require many tiny but vital steps.

It's important to note that recognising these states might sound simple, but it can be difficult to do, especially at first. The very fact that we are in those states means we've lost our capacity for rational, logical thinking and problem-solving. So this process of noticing and recognising is something we must practise with curiosity and a lot of self-compassion. It might look like learning to notice the early warning signs, or being able to reflect later,

'Well, gee whiz, no wonder that argument went nowhere, I was totally outside my Window of Tolerance!' We actually use language that reflects this all the time – 'I was out of my head' or 'I lost my mind'. In fact, we speak from our body in so many ways: 'Keep your chin up!'; 'I've got a gut feeling'; 'I was weak at the knees'; 'It's on the tip of my tongue'; 'I'm so heavy-hearted'. Keeping up the self-compassion as we get to know the way our nervous system operates is at the heart of this invitation.

I also want to acknowledge that some people live in circumstances where their safety and freedom is very compromised. In this situation, teaching your nervous system to feel safe isn't appropriate or even possible. These are situations of crisis, though, and need other resources, such as professional counselling, income support and perhaps medical care. There are some suggestions for crisis support in the resources section (see page 258).

Applying creative first aid habits to your day are micro steps that can add up to a big difference in regulating your nervous system. Inch by inch, we are stepping the stairs towards our home, that window of comfort and tolerance where we can feel a sense of safekeeping, curiosity, play and compassion. This is the intention of self-care.

Radical rest, self-care and self-soothing

For us at MakeShift, the meaning of self-care is an act or practice that works to offset, influence and respond to the emotional responses of our nervous system in ways that help shift us into our Window of Tolerance.

It's not, as magazines and social media might suggest, a day at the spa, or some fancy moisturiser. Those things are nice, and probably more in the camp of self-soothing, which is important, too. More on that soon.

We 'enter the chat' on self-care with some caution. The term itself can induce eye-rolls, and the exhausting sense that there is yet another thing we should be doing along with offsetting our carbon footprint, baking sourdough, inventing a side hustle and hashtag-doing-what-you-love.

It's also become a concept that is wholly entangled with privilege, reserved only for wealthy (and usually white) women with spare cash and time. While we acknowledge that the political and systemic influences on self-care are problematic, we also believe it is a right of every single person to have time and space to tend to themselves. The fact we've created cultural norms where that exists only for some is indeed a big freaking problem.

In any case, self-care in our language does not mean the performative and well-funded actions of the worried well. It's the deeply vital act of restoration and rest that is the fundamental need of every single human, however we can make that happen. Systems and politics are working strongly against large numbers of people finding breathing room for this. Understandably, collective resentment of even the suggestion of self-care is a boiling pot of water on the stovetop of public conversation.

One of the almightiest barriers that seems to face people in efforts to mend their wellbeing is the idea of taking time to rest and practise self-care. The all-encompassing social programming that wires us to see rest as laziness, idleness as indulgence, and self-care as selfish, can be laid squarely at the feet of capitalism, which demands an at-once impossible seesaw of productivity and work, and consumption. Wearing busyness as a badge of honour is almost a requirement.[9]

To rest is to step away from the machine of relentless work. It is to daydream, to play; it is restorative. Artist, poet and activist Tricia Hersey speaks of the act of rest as an act of care for our future self, one that creates room in our lives for inventing things, creating connections and finding answers.[10]

Self-care and self-soothing: not the same thing!

We have become so deskilled in the practice of true, deep rest and self-care that its faster but less effective cousin, self-soothing, has replaced it. If you're not familiar with self-soothing, it's where Netflix, a few wines and a bit of scrolling mindlessly on social media come into the picture. These things help us to tune out, not in. They can serve a useful purpose and are completely fine in moderation, but often don't prompt much of a shift in the way we are actually feeling.

The truth is, we need both: self-care and self-soothing. To actually shift from one state to another, we need to go a little deeper, we need to practise self-care regularly. Sometimes this can feel a little harder. We are tired and it can be easier to scroll Instagram than to go for a walk in nature or do some expressive writing, which would actually calm our nervous system. Just like getting into a pool on a cool day, or doing a gym workout, we might not feel like doing it but we never regret it. It's invigorating, replenishing and restorative, and we emerge from every act of self-care feeling different from before.

Author Charlotte Wood explores this idea and its connection to consumerism and our culture of immediate feedback in a wonderful essay titled 'Reading Isn't Shopping'. 'We've been slowly but thoroughly trained to see the world in terms of its capacity to please us,' Wood says. 'Nowhere have I been asked to rate anything on its capacity to make me uncomfortable, to unnerve or challenge or confuse me. And the prompt for rating, the anxious question, "Did you like it?" arrives moments after the "consumption" takes place. What if I were asked to think about what I've experienced and respond in a month, a year, a decade? It's unthinkable.'[11]

Practising self-soothing instead of self-care can also dampen our ability to experience shock, dismay and disgust. If we numb and soothe ourselves to the flavour of these experiences, we also numb the moments of delight and joy, and those tiny sparks of awe. It's why including some proper, meaningful self-care habits is essential. These habits keep our nervous system steady, and are a space to practise imperfection, uncertainty, play, flow, disgust, delight and all those vital things. Feeling the full range of human experiences is important for a healthy, thriving life and also skills us in being able to live among people and ideas we don't necessarily agree with.

Self-care encompasses the protective habits that help to calm and regulate our nervous system. If you explore the range of prescriptions at the back of this book (starting on page 158), from micro relief practices to recharging activities and habits that restore us, then over time, you'll have a set of available, familiar tools to use whenever you need them. This encourages resilience and enables us to have some degree of control over our emotional response and state. Ultimately, self-care can become a non-negotiable part of our everyday life, not something we add to our future to-do list, to tick off one day, if we ever have the time. Creative first aid creates space in our life to practise learning, playing, failing, and being shocked, delighted and full of joy.

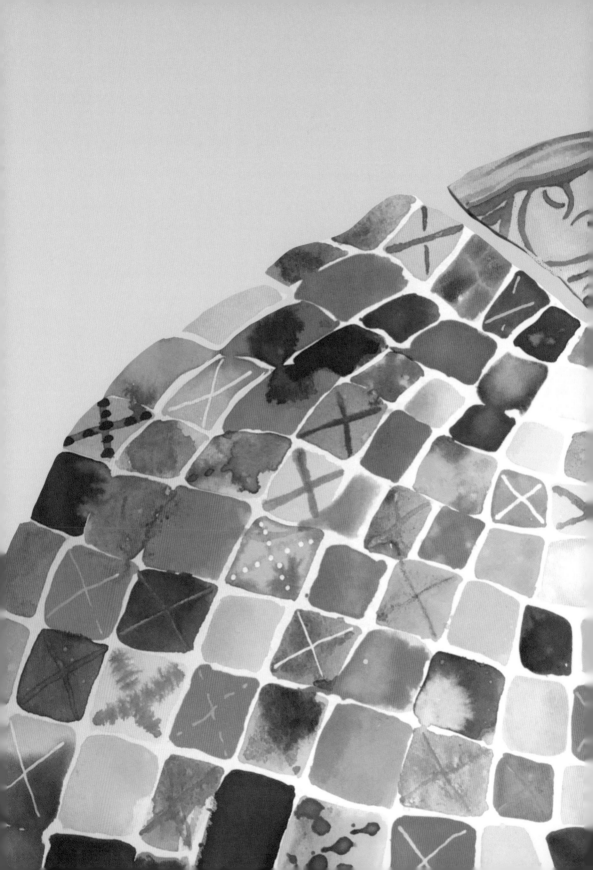

For me, this work feels like a constant and ongoing reflective process. I now rarely find myself in that once-familiar and regular fight/flight state of extremely agitated anxiety, waves of visceral and overwhelming dread pulsing throughout my body, the heaviness in my chest making it hard to breathe. And I have my trusty creative friends to thank for this: my piano, my drawing pencils, my dog-walk loop, my playlists. And it's not always comfortable or pretty. But I take my 'medicine' thinking, 'Okay, well I better take my stupid body for a stupid walk and it's hard and I hate everything and what is the point, but I'll do it anyway because I trust the other versions of myself that have figured out that this helps.' And it always does help.

One vital legacy from experiencing seismic vicarious trauma when I was 23 has been the deep understanding that giving yourself permission to restore and reset and rest and build up mental reserves is just a non-negotiable part of being human.

It's why I would look around at the other mothers, when we were all blindly and tentatively stepping through those first months in that first year of motherhood, and wonder why I didn't find it as hard as everyone else to hand my beloved baby over to her father, or a very generous friend, so that I could have a swim, or a half-hour alone, or a night out, or a rest. I understood that this is what could make the difference between 'good' and loving mothering, and 'barely making it through' mothering, although this felt like a deficit and flaw at the time.

It means that to rest, to play, to take time away from work and caring responsibility and studying and volunteering is a radical act. We are doing it against a powerful wave of visible and covert messaging telling us this makes us lazy or selfish or indulgent. We might bump up against these messages, either in our own head or from the world around us, but what's important is to notice those thoughts – *Oh, there you are* – that deep wiring of relentless productivity, and keep inching forward towards self-care.

Engaging in self-care is a way to untangle the tentacles of productivity that modern life has wrapped around us. It helps us remember that we have value, no matter what. Witnessing people deny themselves care and become overwhelmed with guilt and shame for prioritising their own needs is the most heartbreaking thing I experience in my work. To me, taking time to rest, to play and to administer self-care is a radical act. Sharing this belief is part of the reason we wrote this book.

Proper self-care unfolds into community care

The conversation about self-care is noisy. Critics say that self-care has become the realm of narcissistic navel-gazing, while at the same time so many vulnerable people in our community are isolated and without support. At MakeShift, we see self-care as a key step on the path towards greater community care. Community care is the way people are able to show up and support each other in challenging times. A lot of our work delivering creative first aid programs in disaster-affected communities is all about this. Local government partners have identified that a connected community, built on relationships born during times of safe stability, is essential for being able to respond well in a crisis. If there's trust, familiarity, shared experiences, and the safety to be vulnerable, our communities are stronger, more resilient, more able to band together and leap into action for each other when a crisis is on the doorstep.

Without caring for ourselves first, we can't provide community care and support others around us. Fit your own oxygen mask before you help others, as they say. To be able to show up for other people – our family, our community, our workplace – requires us to be in a regulated, rested state.

Dysregulation makes us poorer judges of others' intentions and behaviours – seeing a slight sideways glance as an attack, misreading an unreturned message as a clear act of rejection. This can tip people into incorrectly labelling every difficult experience as trauma, or every disagreement as a toxic conflict. A whole community of dysregulated people will mean a whole community of people at odds with each other, feeling angry, fearful, critical and quick to judge.

The practice of meaningful, regulating self-care is how we grow and cultivate empathy. Self-care shifts us inch by inch towards that window of grounded mindfulness, meaning we are able to own our responses, and see where we are reacting out of ego or shame. Outside our Window of Tolerance, we might push the words of others through a sausage machine of meaning-making so it comes out as perceived criticism, instead of actually hearing the words of others from a place of peace and separation. Self-care is the soil in which the seeds of social connection grow.

Individuals who take care of their psychological needs – through creative first aid – are going to have a far greater capacity to care for each other, to collectively respond and offer help with compassion, understanding and generosity.

We are hardwired for co-regulation

Humans are hardwired for connection. It's a well-established fact in psychology. Maslow's hierarchy of needs, the model for understanding motivations for human behaviour, points to love and belonging as central to a thriving life.[12] We have always lived in organised communities, seeking out relationships and forming groups in order to be seen and to relate to those around us in safe and rewarding ways. It is the absence of this that can cause so much internal and social distress, loneliness and psychological pain.

While we talk a lot in this book about self-regulation, it does not happen in a vacuum. We look for thousands of non-verbal cues from other people, through eye contact, tone of voice and body language, to signal whether we are safe or not in their company. Having the capacity to self-regulate is important, but this works completely in tandem with co-regulation. Think about the way we are tuned in to non-verbal cues, the way babies respond to skin contact, the way we adjust our voice to speak with an upset child, or the way we initiate direct eye contact when a friend shares some challenging news.

The Maharishi Effect famously measured the stress levels of people close to a large group meditating together[13] and found a significant decrease in cortisol (stress hormones) just from being in proximity to others in a state of mindful bliss. This research led to intentional group meditation being used in high-crime communities in urban cities in the US, which resulted in a drop in crime and violent incidents.[14]

Loneliness has become a critical public health issue, and in fact has been acknowledged as being more dangerous to our health than smoking.[15] Covid-19 and lockdowns, over years, has had a far-reaching impact on our community connections.[16] While smartphones and social media can give us the illusion of being connected, meaningful relationships with others continue to be elusive and out of reach for many. To change this requires both a collective normalising of self-care as essential for our lives, and an understanding that community and social connection is a fundamental human need.

If we are feeling calm and grounded (i.e. inside our Window of Tolerance), we are primed to connect safely, compassionately and more easily. Creative practices can help encourage that sense of rested regulation. Through the workshops we run, Lizzie and I have witnessed time and time again that the motivation to open up, reach out and curiously engage comes when people are doing something they enjoy.

This story comes to life beautifully in my chat with Jono Brand, artistic director of the Captain Starlight Program whom we met in Chapter 2 (see page 64). He talks about his early days as Captain Starlight, walking into a large ward room with six beds divided by flimsy curtains, literal barriers to connection. He would say to his co-captain, 'By the time we leave we want all those curtains open, and everyone to be talking to each other.' Through their considered, playful clowning expertise, riffing off each other and making the kids the centre of the play, this would become reality in lightning-quick time, and by the time Jono and his co-captain left the ward, kids and parents would be talking and laughing, swapping stories and numbers.

We can't fake this type of connection, or put it in a pill. If we don't receive it, we will feel an absence in our lives, sometimes in a way we can't put our finger on. If wellbeing is defined as having agency over how our nervous system responds to tricky times, then being well also means being in a place ripe for connection – open, curious, grounded, clear, available for nuance and disagreement in a way that doesn't prick at our sense of safety.

✳ **Field note** – Restoring things, restoring me: Leanne's story

Leanne was a police officer for 14 years. After working on a high volume of domestic violence cases, she left the force due to post-traumatic stress disorder (PTSD). We met Leanne in 2020 when she joined our eight-week ReMind course. Three years later, Lizzie caught up with her on Zoom.

Leanne arrives on Zoom in perpetual motion. She carries her laptop as she walks around the house, first to her lounge room, then through the kitchen to tend to the clawing cat at her screen door. All I can see is the ceiling and it's making me giddy.

'Sorry about that,' she says, as she settles into a comfy chair to tell me her story. 'I've walked seven kilometres today. I walk every day. I have to, or my mind starts racing too fast. I also need to restore furniture every day or my mind gets out of hand.

'Early on in my career, about ten years in, I was in a team that had a reputation for attracting murders, deceased estates and pretty bad jobs. The policy back then was that if you attended five "bad jobs" over a certain period of time, the duty officer would check on your welfare. I guess this was a quasi-system of care, but what happened was a duty officer came up to me and said, "I'm supposed to check on you, but you're okay, aren't you, mate?" I had no choice but to say yes.

'But one day I couldn't cope any more. It wasn't from a bad job; it was the accumulation of all of the work and the culture within the force. I just broke down. I was working at the counter and I just burst into tears. I couldn't stop crying and began rocking back and forth. I tried really hard to pull myself together, to just brush it off, but I rapidly declined and ended up leaving the force. It's been a long road since then. Getting involved in MakeShift and engaging in a creative practice really set me on a pathway to where I am now, and significantly improved my symptoms of PTSD.

'At the beginning I was so challenged by creativity, so frustrated by it. But I'm pretty stubborn, so I kept trying and eventually, while drawing, I experienced that feeling of getting lost in a process – it felt so freeing. It just opened my mind right up. Now, I can't stop, it snaps me back into the present and stops me from feeling overwhelmed. You can't sand furniture and be thinking about how crap you feel, or what you're going to do with your life. You have to be in the moment or you'll damage what you're working on and probably accidentally sand your own hands!'

Leanne walks down the hallway into a large room. The camera eventually lands on a beautiful chest of oak drawers. 'This,' she beams, 'is what calms my mind, keeps me going. This is my therapy. Restoring an old piece of furniture into a new version of itself is exactly what I have done to myself.'

Finding what works for you

The invitation here for getting to know your nervous system brings us back to the five foundational elements of creative first aid. In the same way that we apply them when we start a new creative activity, such as journal writing or collage, we can apply them in a really useful way to exploring our own nervous system.

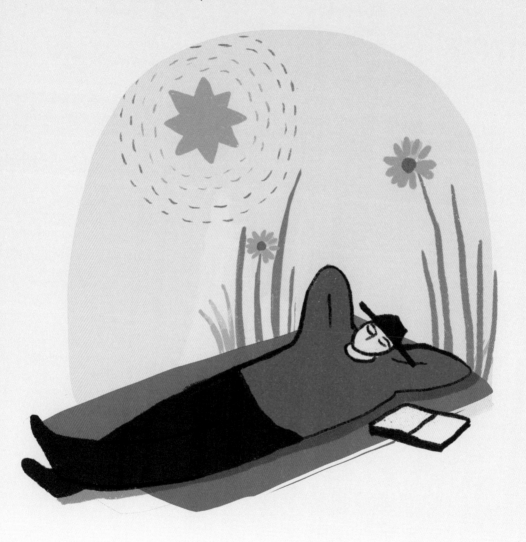

The five elements of creative first aid

Starting with **self-compassion**, use the Window of Tolerance tool to begin tuning in to the messages your body is giving you. Notice patterns, without judgement.

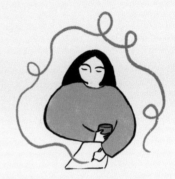

Be **curious** about noticing those early signs of inching out of your Window of Tolerance. They are unconscious and will lack logic sometimes, instead being physical sensations in your body.

Take note of how building habits out of acts of play, joy, rest and restoration can increase a sense of safety and **safekeeping**.

Try out some practices that bring you into a state of **playfulness**. Be curious in noticing whether they create any micro shifts back towards grounded rest and digest.

Slowly a plan emerges, **inch by inch**, of habits – even ones that just take a few minutes – that become non-negotiable parts of your day to keep you in your Window of Tolerance as much as possible.

The Creative Prescriptions starting on page 158 are a guide to exploring more grounding prescriptions for recharge and restoration, which can form a really vital antidote to nervous system dysregulation. Start small and be kind to yourself.

✳ **Field note** – Weaving towards safety: Michele's story

Michele Elliot contacted MakeShift in 2015, offering to teach stitching and embroidery. Her workshops were an immediate success – her warm, gentle and calming presence providing the perfect atmosphere for people wanting to learn practices of Indian *kantha*, slow stitching, shibori dyeing, sewing. But Michele had overcome a lot to get to this point. She had become ill while travelling through Nepal with friends in April 2015, and was near Kathmandu when the 7.8 magnitude Gorkha earthquake hit.

'I woke up to what I thought was the sound of dogs running around on the roof of my hotel. I opened my eyes and there was plaster falling on my face and I somehow managed to sit up. It was an earthquake. A big one. I got myself up and to the doorway, then one of the porters came and helped me out. By that stage, the whole ground beneath us was moving like this rolling wave. We got outside and I was quite delirious, I think, so I was laid down on the ground, and then shortly afterwards came this absolutely massive aftershock. It was terrifying.

'Places that we'd been to just days before were completely obliterated. What happened over those days, the scale of the loss of life was devastating. We were eventually evacuated – it was a huge rescue operation.

We were so grateful for all of that, it was quite surreal. Months later, back in Australia, I had another bout of flu and I literally collapsed. I woke up one morning and couldn't get out of bed. I looked at my hands and they were shaking, quite noticeably trembling. That went on for a couple of days, so I got myself to my doctor. It was sort of this delayed response to what happened in Nepal, about five months after. I'd only ever known about PTSD in terms of people like soldiers that have been through the experience of war or people that have lived through domestic violence. I'd never really thought about it in relation to the earthquake.

'In some ways I feel like that trembling was a manifestation of the earthquake – that I'd kind of carried something of that shaking back with me inside my body. It was like an eruption inside me, and it took me a while to realise what was going on. It was a kind of strange physical manifestation of what had actually happened.'

While Michele's mind consciously and rationally understood that she had lived through a traumatic earthquake, she figured that because she was now home and safe, she should be fine. But her body felt something different. She was literally reliving the physical tremors and quaking of that experience in terrifyingly physical ways, a very visible nervous system response that didn't make sense in a logical, rational way. After she found her hands shaking out of control, months after the earthquake, she sought help through her local doctor.

'I'd been talking to my GP one day about the changes that I wanted to make. She's really involved in what's called "social prescribing", and said to me, "Do you know about this organisation called MakeShift? You've got all these things that you can teach people. Why don't you think about connecting with them and doing some work in the community?"

'So I started teaching some community classes, which was such a welcome change from academic teaching, and around the same time became an artist-in-residence at Tender Funerals, an amazing not-for-profit service based in Port Kembla. I held, and still hold, sewing circles there to work with families. The stitching is really about finding ways of learning techniques that will help somebody through that process of grief.

'What happened in becoming involved in these two organisations was it became a way for me to engage with my own practice, as well as to engage with other people and to then create a kind of space for social stitching. It's as much for me as for others, and has become about this space and sense of community where I live and work.'

Michele's journey of healing from the trauma of the earthquake makes this body knowledge about our nervous system come to life. Her body unconsciously called out about what it felt was continuing alarm and danger, shouting at her in a way that demanded instant attention.

Another GP may have gone down the route of prescribing pharmaceuticals, and these might have relieved Michele's physical symptoms. But would this have transformed her life in the way that engaging in creative practices with her community did? Instead, her GP prescribed social connection through creative practice. She heard Michele's interest in working in her community and understood that in order to treat her PTSD, Michele needed to make some life changes.

'For me, this has been about being present in the place where we live, my home. Through making those connections, there's been a kind of grounding that I think is really about healing. As an artist, I already had this habit of repetitive practice to turn to. It was widening out to be about working with others that made the difference, but it all starts with practice. There's something about building a practice that really lets you have that time with yourself. If it's something that's new to you, then often repetitive activities are a really great way to start with that. A beautiful ease and familiarity happen when you practise something every day.'

Michele certainly wandered far from home. In a literal sense she travelled from Australia all the way to Nepal and nearly didn't return. She also wandered far from her sense of safety and groundedness, from her Window of Tolerance. Thankfully, she found her way back, in all senses. By taking each moment as it came, being curious and getting to know what her body was telling her, she was able to reach out and begin healing. Like the threads she works with every day, she wove herself deeply into her community and through this found peace.

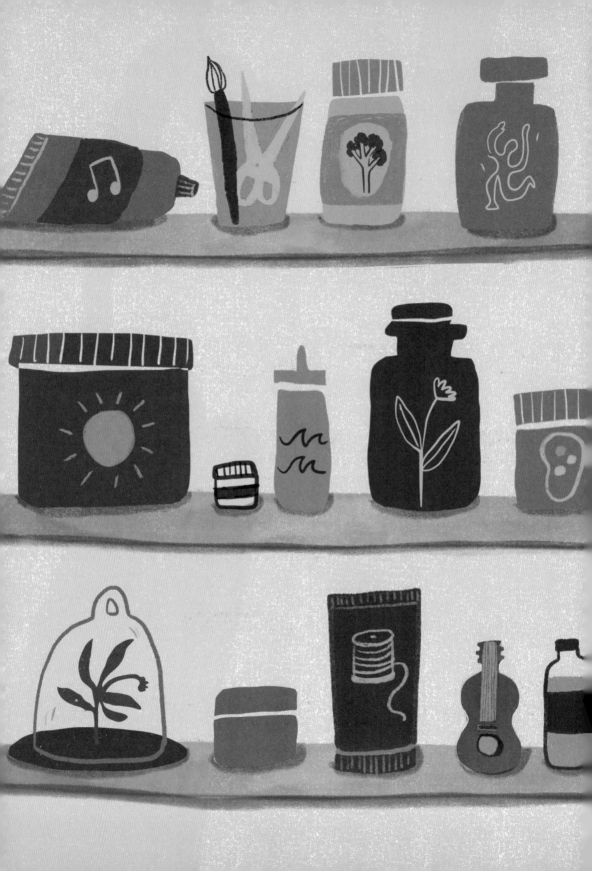

CHAPTER 5

The Creative Dispensary

Welcome to the Creative Dispensary. This dispensary is a carefully curated group of 50 prescriptions that have been tried and tested by us as well as people we've worked with. They have come to us from far and wide, offered as accessible remedies for nervous system care by artists, musicians, gardeners, yoga teachers, a midwife, writers and ecologists, and directly from a decade of working in creative prescribing. We hope they are as effective for you as they have been for thousands of MakeShift workshop attendees. The best way in is one foot forward and a sprinkle of curiosity.

These practices can be done at home, in your office, on a train or even a plane, and they don't require you to spend a bunch of money. Some of them might require items you don't have on hand, but don't worry, you can always get creative and improvise! Each activity is designed as a universal invitation and embodies – as our friend and collage artist Angie Cass calls it – the democracy of craft. In almost all instances, there's little more required than everyday household items such as paper, pens, scissors and maybe some string or yarn.

You are your own guide through this process – be open-armed, curious and compassionate. It's about knowing yourself, and getting to know yourself, in a giant act of play and discovery. Don't forget to apply the five elements of creative first aid that we talked about on pages 35–49: safety, playfulness, inch by inch, curiosity and self-compassion.

Know thyself

Way back in the olden days, otherwise known as 2001, *Amélie* was a wildly popular French film. Set in Paris, it's the tale of a young woman, full of quirks and oddly endearing traits, who finds love unexpectedly.

Each character in the film is introduced by a narrator, with a short list of their likes and dislikes. Amélie's father, for example, likes peeling off large strips of wallpaper, lining up all his shoes and polishing them, and emptying out his toolbox, cleaning it out, and putting everything back in again. He dislikes clingy wet swimming trunks, scornful looks at his sandals, and peeing next to someone in a public urinal.

Each of these lists so beautifully capture the essence of the character, allowing the audience to build empathy for them immediately. It also reveals a kind of universal truth that each and every person has a unique set of likes and dislikes, and knowing them about yourself is an essential part of how to live a good life.

In BP (before pandemic) times, we ran all of our workshops and events in real life, with people, face to face and in 3D. Back then, Karen Yello, our wonderful friend and the wisest of humans, assisted us by bringing what we call the 'zhoosh'. Like a whimsical fairy, Karen would place disco balls on trees, crystals on windowsills, crocheted blankets on people's knees, warm lamps where the light was too bright, and cushions under bums.

Prescription

In the spirit of both Karen, and the film *Amélie*, we invite you to create your own love and loathe list.

Grab some paper and a pen, and spend a few minutes reflecting on these things, writing them down. Try to make them small: for example, 'I love clicking together sealable sandwich bags, and the sensation of cat paws walking on my arm.' While the big stuff is important, it can activate us and stress us out, so keep this list about the little things, such as, 'I loathe the sound of nails down a blackboard.' This list might change every single day.

This is like a little warm-up for starting a voyage into creative first aid. It can remind you that you do have gut instinct, inner wisdom, and curiosity to play. It can also affirm the fact that you are unique and interesting, and that finding new and fun things to love and loathe is a process that can continue every future day of your life.

Time for a little self-audit

No doubt you already have some strategies, habits and things you do to keep yourself steady. Most people do. Maybe it's walking a beloved dog each morning, or doing a crossword. Going to the gym, or doing some meditation. Maybe your go-to strategies for when things are overwhelming don't serve you so well – doom-scrolling on social media is so tempting, but rarely leaves us feeling restored and rejuvenated. Throwing yourself into work might be a distraction, but also a pattern that leaves little time for restoration.

Reflecting on the protective self-care strategies that you already have is useful. It can help highlight and bring clarity about where there are gaps. This is especially useful in thinking about the ways you experience moving out of your Window of Tolerance. For people who tend to shift into that very heightened, activated state of fight/flight, it means ensuring that some potent, sensory practices make up part of your set of self-care strategies. Or if you find yourself inching more often toward the freeze/collapse state, some gentle, soothing actions to wake up your system will be helpful. Consider this a nudge to take a moment to conduct an audit on yourself. Knock, knock! The auditors are here!

You can do this audit by asking yourself the following questions:

* What's something you do each week that makes you feel good?
* What are you already doing that helps you stay in your Window of Tolerance? Do those things add to restoring you, or do they cost you?[1]
* Is there something you thought you might want to do but has never quite stuck? What made it hard to keep up? (A good check is to see if self-criticism was the reason.) Were you too focused on being really good at it?
* Where is there a window of five minutes in your day? Fifteen minutes? An hour?

You may realise you already have familiar practices that can go into your creative first aid kit. Write them down! You might also have the sorts of materials you will need lying around. Go find them!

Your own nervous system

You are the only you, and so figuring out what is going to work for you is a personal journey. It's time to reflect on the Window of Tolerance tool.

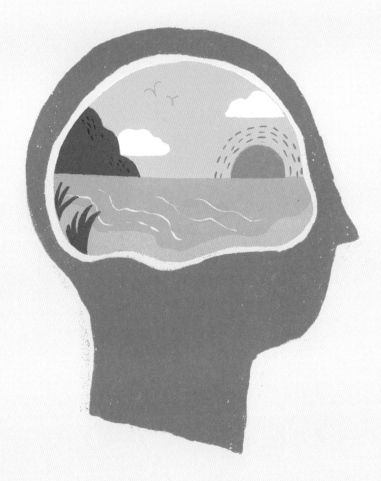

To begin this project of data collection on yourself, again, we go through a process of powerful reflective questions. See if you can do this every day for a week. Make some notes about what you notice.

Remember that what is happening with your nervous system doesn't need to be labelled 'good' or 'bad', it just is. It's an unconscious process, and this is the beginning of taking a little control.

Start with the Body Weather Mapping prescription on page 194.

* Notice if you feel a sense of being in the present. Do you feel connected to your body?
* Are there different physical sensations you notice? Tightness or lightness, for example?
* Do you feel at 'home' (safe, comfortable, able to let your mind wander)?
* Do you feel rational, logical and able to solve problems creatively? Or do you feel a sense of worry and are you thinking catastrophic thoughts?
* Do you feel dread or nothing at all? Is it hard to even concentrate on these questions?

This process can help locate yourself in your Window of Tolerance. Make a note of where you think you are, and by repeating that over numerous days, you will start to build a picture of how your nervous system is functioning. Self-compassion and curiosity are your friends here.

If you really struggle with naming or noticing these experiences, it's okay. This process can be difficult to start with. Instead, it can be an opportunity to try out some practices like the prescriptions we offer in this book and see what happens. See how they make you feel, or what sensations they provide.

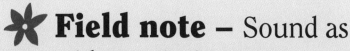 **Field note** – Sound as an antidote: Lisa's story

Lisa is in her mid-forties, has two kids and has a penchant for musical theatre. She was a weapons trainer for the police force for 20 years. She has witnessed more than most people ever will and heard sounds that most people shouldn't hear.

'One day I cracked. It had been building in me for a while. I felt myself starting to shut down, and then the trauma psych was called in.

'I loved teaching people things, and joined the force because my parents wouldn't let me join the military, so the decision was kind of made for me. I didn't want to be bored. Also, I love a uniform! That appealed to me. Eliminating deciding what to wear each day was just one less decision to make. I think this is why creativity has really worked for me. Two things changed my life: movement and sound. Discovering those things in the MakeShift program, and also in musical theatre, changed my life, as well as mantras.'

This really means a lot, given Lisa's background with the police and how her nervous system has been hardwired for danger. Listening to certain mantras helps prepare Lisa for anything, sometimes just feeling brave enough to leave the house.

'With creativity, there is no right or wrong, there's no policy or procedure. Creativity helps you break the cycle by letting you make mistakes and that feels okay. It gives you permission to try and gives you back power. I guess all that stuff is tied up in this idea of critical decision-making, where you just can't afford to make mistakes. So yeah, wearing a uniform and playing the ukulele are like an antidote to stressful decisions! Not that I do them together!

'It took me a while to get to this point, but I was curious and kept trying things. I think that being creative calms you down, it makes you feel lighter, not so soul heavy. The more I do it, the easier it is and then it's like my body remembers what it feels like to be in that space of being creative and I can start to take myself back to that feeling of being in that space, even when I'm not actually doing the practice. The after-effect is sometimes just as beneficial. It's like tapping in to the mind–body spot and lingering there.

'I was a cop in the force for 20 years, I had no relationship with, or understanding of, rhythm, vibration or sound. But it's been one thing that's saved me in really dark times over and over again. Certain frequencies and sounds can literally feel like a tonic on my nervous system and calm me down in minutes, and noise, such as traffic, machinery and the fast pace of life can completely derail me.'

What do you need and what do you want?

Think about what you need for yourself. Do you need first aid right now? Or are you a little further along and need some deeper, longer-lasting medicine?

It's worth mentioning here that sometimes what you want isn't the same as what you need. Exploring creative first aid requires you to stretch and challenge yourself, just as going to therapy or asking for help does. There will be discomfort, but ultimately these are really important and positive steps to take outside your comfort zone.

You'll find three types of remedies in the Creative Prescriptions on pages 160 to 251.

1. Remedies for relief

These practices are designed to be short, quick and powerful, and can act as a reboot for when we are moving outside our Window of Tolerance. Each activity can be completed in around five to ten minutes, and might be called for just before you have to give a big, scary work presentation, or after a very difficult phone call, or just when you're feeling caught up in a noisy fuzz of fear and stress.

On the surface, these practices can seem rather simple, even inconsequential. Just remember that the goal is to tap in to your body's unconscious response, giving it a message that you are safe, it's okay to relax. These remedies for relief are great to practise again and again. Over time they can make a big difference, as our nervous system learns to recognise these practices as cues of safety and regulation.

2. Remedies for recharging

Once you are out of the emergency zone and feeling more regulated, you are able to engage in practices that are a little longer and more involved. These activities require slightly more time and preparation – some of them ask for some materials to assemble – and are great for when you notice warning signs that you are shifting outside your Window of Tolerance (see page 121). They can still fit into a lunchbreak, or those quiet moments before a big day. They are not designed to blow out your schedule in ways that create more stress.

Recharging practices might grow to become little anchors you can drop down regularly. They are for when you might start to recognise those early signs that you are moving out towards the edges of your Window of Tolerance. Early intervention is the best intervention! Like sunscreen, they can become a regular application that protects our emotional state from swinging into chaos that feels out of our control.

3. Remedies for restoration

The last collection of prescriptions are designed to be restorative. The activities are deeper and longer; they are ones that you can get lost in, that help you find your state of flow. Like taking a course of antibiotics, the impact of these activities continues long after you have completed them.

These practices can create rhythms for when you are grounded, connected and able to be immersed in the fun of play. They are for a free afternoon, or day off, or an evening at home. Many of them are an invitation to fling yourself into the nearest patch of nature, wherever you can find it. (This is so often the answer, really.)

As you experiment with the remedies, we encourage you to figure out which ones work for you and then build your own kit of practices. Once you are familiar with them, you can return to them again and again, without having to think too hard. When you play and discover a medium that you enjoy – drawing, perhaps – it can be helpful to create a little art station where you keep your pens and paper, to make it easy to return to. Making a space in your home dedicated to creativity can be a really powerful act of permission, ensuring that you are centring your own self-care.

Hurrah for habits

They say it takes 66 days to form a new habit. A habit is a regular routine of behaviour, one that tends to occur subconsciously. Habits are actions we take regardless of the weather.

We suggest going through these remedies and finding a handful that you really connect with. Maybe try something every day for a week and see how it makes you feel. The strength of many of these practices is going to be felt over time.

We invite you to practise these prescriptions as habits, even when you are comfortably inside your Window of Tolerance (see page 121). By becoming familiar with these activities, you can turn to them without too much effort when life feels hard.

The other important thing to say here is that when we find ourselves in lots of intense, dysregulated moments, it's often because life is stressful. Whether it's related to work, relationships, finances or health, there are plenty of times when it feels like our last priority is being creative. For some of us, this is All the Time. It's How Things Are. That is hard, tricky and exhausting. This is the time to inch towards more deep self-care, not less. It's the time for as many regulation practices that we can trust and know help us, even if it's just a few minutes of them at a time. Once we find a set of practices ready to apply in all sorts of moments, the greatest gift we can give ourselves is making them a habit. Walk when it's sunny, or rainy, windy or cold. Walk to wander and return home. And the more we do that, the easier it is to do.

Like brushing your teeth

In our programs and sessions, we often talk about 'brushing your teeth', because it's an act of self-care that we do every day, usually even twice a day. We don't psych ourselves up to do it. We don't go through the list of pros and cons in our head.

Ideally this is the way we fit some of our self-care, self-restoration habits into our day, too. If we do them enough times, we don't need to think too hard about them. Swirling in a state of activated fight or flight is a really hard time to think logically about the steps required to do something helpful. In these states, logic and rational thought are not available, so we can only really turn to what is familiar and nearby. Having developed a practice as a habit means we can turn to it without too much effort and thought.

On their own, some of these prescriptions will be nice to do. Some of them might be something you do just once, and say, 'Well, that was lovely.' The richness of these prescriptions comes with repetition, forming a habit. That's when we have – as the scientists say – data to reflect on. How did you feel after doing this activity once? We get better at knowing what a practice gives to us when we have done it a bunch of times and can more quickly access the effect of the experience because of the familiar sensation, the muscle memory, of having done it before.

So here is your invitation to explore and try and taste, but if you find something that nourishes you, do it again! It can be magical to discover that one little practice, like going for a walk or making a collage, can set you up for limitless possibilities of creative discovery, of wonder and replenishment.

A hot tip for amping up new habits is called habit stacking.[2] This concept invites you to take a habit you already have, such as brushing your teeth or making a coffee in the morning, and stack another new habit on it, so that they happen together. The goal is to then keep this up as a regular action that you do, irrespective of your feelings or motivation.

Motivation is a tricky hook to hang behaviour change on. Many exercise instructors now reject the concept of motivation being part of fitness. They note that if we wait for motivation to start doing something, we might be waiting a while. Instead, we should trust in the impact and benefit that we have felt before, and just turn up. Do it anyway. Do it from a place of self-compassion, but also curiosity.

We've also included some Treatment Plans (see pages 252–55), a collection of creative prescriptions designed to build a habit of drawing, nature connection or creative movement. Of course, you are always free to choose your own adventure.

Enjoy, and keep yourself safe while you stretch, flex and play with your own creativity.

Creative
Prescriptions

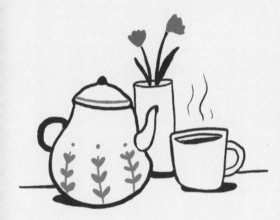

Relief
remedies

Recharge remedies

Restoration remedies

Relief

Five Senses Reboot

MEDIUM

Movement

TIME NEEDED

1–2 minutes

MATERIALS

● Your five senses

This practice of quick and instant grounding has been around for a long time, so long we can't recall where we learnt it or who taught it to us! It is a fast and impactful grounding technique for moments when you are feeling completely overwhelmed. By tuning in to each sense, we signal to our nervous system that it's okay to calm and soften, to slow our breathing down, to really pay attention to the detail of sight, sound, touch, smell and taste. Saying out loud the things identified can work as a mindful regulating action that keeps us in the present.

How to take this dose

✳ Look around you. What are five things you can see? Say them out loud. (For example, clock, picture, glass, plant, door.)

✳ Turn your head. What are four things you can hear? Say them out loud.

✳ Move if you need to. What are three things you can touch?

✳ What are two things you can smell?

✳ What is one thing you can taste?

Benefits

This is a simple nervous system regulation practice used by many clinicians and somatic teachers to bring instant mindful presence to a moment. By engaging with all of our senses in real time, we activate our ventral vagal response (see page 117), which brings us into the present and shifts away from a heightened, activated state.

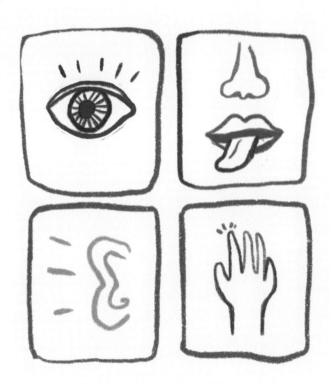

Relief

Compassion Palming

MEDIUM

Movement

TIME NEEDED

1–10 minutes

MATERIALS

● Your body

This practice was gifted to us by our friend Sarah Ball, a trauma-sensitive and mental-health-focused yoga teacher. It's wonderful when you're feeling tender, tired or unsettled, or needing some self-care and self-kindness.

How to take this dose

✱ Rub your palms together until you feel some warmth.

✱ As you feel the warmth build in your hands, take a steady inhalation.

✱ As you exhale, place the palms of your hands over your closed eyes, on the front of your throat, or over your heart.

✱ Pause and feel your own touch and its soothing powers. You can repeat the process for as long as it feels good.

Benefits

Caring physical gestures enable us to shift the idea of self-compassion from a concept to a real-time, tangible action. By stimulating the sensory areas in the palms of your hands, you invoke sensations that can distract a busy mind and regulate your nervous system. Using your breath to regulate and soothe, while also offering yourself the warmth and touch of your own hands, can further assist in calming your nervous system.

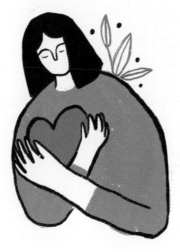

Relief

Write to Release

MEDIUM

Reading &
Writing

TIME NEEDED

5 minutes

MATERIALS

● A timer
● A piece of A4 paper
● A pen

We learnt this practice from working with award-winning young adult fiction author and writing teacher Helena Fox. Helena speaks beautifully and authentically about the way writing can provide many forms of self-care: release, reflection, tools of observation, play, etc.

How to take this dose

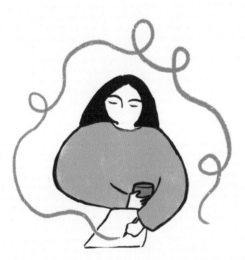

✱ Choose one of these words as a prompt to get started: pulse, shine, run, grow, safe. If you're inspired by anything else around you, you can use that as a prompt instead!

✱ Set a timer, and try to write continuously for 5 minutes without reading or editing what you have written.

✱ Take a minute to read what you've written. Something within it might give you a jolt of inspiration to do something else. Maybe you want to keep writing. Or not.

Benefits

Writing in this way helps empty the mind and release unspoken sensations and feelings. The process of writing activates different parts of our brain than talking does. Writing for release can feel like closing all the tabs on your computer, or sweeping the floor, leaving you feeling more energised, calmer and clearer.

Relief

Mindful Mindless Mark Making

MEDIUM

Mark Making

TIME NEEDED

1–5 minutes

MATERIALS

- A piece of A4 or A5 paper
- Something to make a mark with (a pencil, Sharpie, texta, etc.)

Melinda Young is a contemporary jeweller, educator, maker, beachcomber and craft lover. She is the kind of person who is never without a project; her hands are always busy making. Mel is a creative facilitator for the MakeShift ReMind program and has generously gifted us this practice for the book. She has taught us that craft is a reliable companion you can take anywhere.

How to take this dose

Take three big breaths, in and out. Notice the tension you might feel in different parts of your body.

Sit comfortably, with the paper in front of you, and close your eyes.

Start, feeling with your fingers, making repetitive marks on the page in rows. The marks could be lines, dots, swirls, arcs, circles, squiggles – whatever feels good. There is no wrong way to do this.

When you finish a row, move down and across to do another row. If you notice your thoughts drifting to, 'Oh no, I've messed it up! I've done it wrong! This is going terribly,' let them go by, and keep going. Keep making marks.

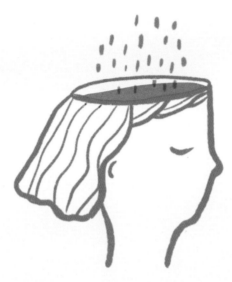

If you realise you are tensely gripping onto your pen, take a second to loosen your grip, and take a breath. Slow down – there is no rush. See if you can fill the page.

If you are feeling a little calmer, grab another page and keep going!

Benefits

This activity helps bring us into the present and slow down. It is especially useful on those days when you feel far away from your goals or from yourself. When we slow down and make repeated patterns, we activate the parasympathetic nervous system, basically where we find our Window of Tolerance (see page 121). Repetition, such as making marks on a page over and over, also helps cultivate a mindful flow state and provide a framework for starting a meditation process. It reminds us that we can get through the day, or the week; we just need to take things one step at a time.

Relief

Four Faces

MEDIUM

Mark Making

TIME NEEDED

Start with 2 minutes

MATERIALS

- **A piece of A4 paper**
- **Something to draw with (crayons, textas, Sharpies, pastels; whatever you have on hand)**

This exercise is adapted from illustrator and graphic designer Marcelo Baez and his drawing workshops at Makeshift. Marcelo has facilitated these workshops for diverse audiences – from a room full of insurance brokers to people engaging in trauma recovery work. His goal is to make each person recognise that they can draw. Faces are everywhere, and this exercise also reminds us of how every different person our eyes fall upon is entirely unique. No two cheeks, eyebrows, teeth, noses, ears, hairstyles or complexions are the same. And that is quite a wonderful thing.

How to take this dose

Start with a blank piece of paper and draw four circles on it. Don't be too precise, they do not need to be perfect.

With the same marker, or a different one, make three quick dashes inside each circle. Make the dashes in each circle different. Again, don't overthink it, there is no wrong way of doing this.

Using as many markers or colours as you like, you now have six marks to spend on each circle, turning it into a face of some kind. You could spend a mark making a pink circle that becomes a tongue. Or a black triangle nostril. Play with expressions. Do the faces look angry? Worried? Scared? Hopeful? Cheeky? Take delight in all the different and funny looks you create. Spend time falling into the activity, colouring in a bow tie or creating wavy curls.

You just drew four faces! And faces are often the scariest things to draw.

Benefits

Drawing as an act of play warms up our creative muscle. It gets us into the zone or flow that promotes a state of mindfulness. By keeping things limited and simple – a circle, a line, six simple marks – we also limit the boundaries of our self-criticism. Can we really be too critical about a face we've drawn that's made of three lines, a circle and some marks that we don't find perfect?

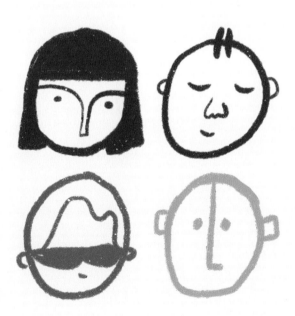

Relief

Blind Contour Drawing

MEDIUM

Mark Making

TIME NEEDED

1–5 minutes

MATERIALS

- A piece of A4 or A5 paper
- Something to make a mark with (a pencil, Sharpie, texta, etc.)
- Access to a mirror, if possible
- A timer

We learnt this practice from visual artist and jeweller Melinda Young. Melinda has been a MakeShift Artist facilitator for many years, bringing her regular visual journalling to life in our programs and workshops.

How to take this dose

Choose something to draw. You could use a mirror to look at your own reflection, or you could be sneaky and draw someone else unawares (on the train, or the bus), or you could pick an object such as a cup, a vase, a plant or a teapot. Make it a fairly simple thing – although faces can be fun!

Sit comfortably so that you can draw on the paper without taking your pen off the page.

Set a timer for about a minute and, without looking at the paper, draw everything you observe. Tune right in to the lines, details and shapes. Remember: don't look and don't lift your pen.

Slow your breathing and focus on drawing what you see and what is there. When you feel like you are finished, check it out. Let laughter out if you have the urge!

If you want to, you can fill in the details with watercolours, collage paper or found materials, paint or even ink. See how the image grows and changes with these added elements.

Benefits

This practice does three important things all at once. Firstly, it brings us smack-bang into the present moment, as we are asking our brain to do something in an unusual way that requires effort. Secondly, it allows us to bypass our inner critic who is telling us that our drawing is bad. Of course, it might be 'bad' – we're not even looking at the paper! Finally, it builds connections with ourselves and those around us. Practising this activity regularly strengthens our ability to embrace imperfection, and enables us to be less attached to our creations.

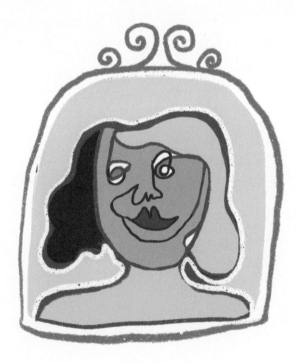

Relief

I Dare You Not to Move

TIME NEEDED

1–5 minutes

MATERIALS

- A few of your favourite songs (and something to listen to them on)

We didn't know we needed a midwife to help us birth this book, but it turns out we did! This practice is dedicated to Marianne Wobcke, a First Nations midwife and trained nurse who specialises in birthing practices and trauma recovery. She came into our lives during the process of writing this book and generously offered to help hold space for us. She frequently peppered our conversations with sentiments like, 'You've got this!' and, 'You're doing so well!' and, 'You're almost there!' After one chat she sent us a playlist to use before we began writing each day and said, 'I dare you not to move.'

How to take this dose

This prescription invites you to think of a few songs that just really make you want to tap your feet, bop your head and move. The drive to dance is hard to ignore! The songs that make you want to move are your own unique callings; everyone will choose different ones.

You might like to put a few of these into a playlist and call it I DARE YOU NOT TO MOVE. Feel free to call it whatever you like.

The intention is that when we need a real reset, when we feel dread pulsing through us, or are worried or sad or overwhelmed, we can listen to these songs and find a sense of release through a few minutes of dancing. Whatever you want to call it, it's an instant discharge of energy through the power of music.

We will quickly find that these few minutes carry us through those waters and we land on a new shore feeling a little different. Dance it out.

Benefits

This is a great activity for when you are very much outside your Window of Tolerance (see page 121), or your anxiety is high and you feel scared and jittery. Basically, it's for when you feel like you need to release some energy.

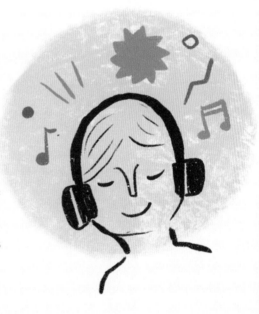

In most indigenous cultures, as well as most evidence-based trauma therapies, movement is considered to be the most crucial action we can take in dealing with those sensations of panic and dread. Dancing, or moving our body in novel and weird ways, disrupts the messages of danger from our amygdala (the part of our brain in charge of emotional processes) to our nervous system, helping it to regulate into a grounded state.

Relief

Owl Eyes

TIME NEEDED

3 minutes

MATERIALS

- Your body

Caitlin and I learnt the practice of owl eyes when we were on a three-day deep nature retreat to learn about the language of birds. It involved a lot of sitting still and quietly in the bush, slowing down and noticing what was happening around us. At one point a teacher took a small group of us aside and taught us the practice of 'owl eyes' as a way of being able to see more widely and notice even more of what was happening around us. It felt like being given a whole new pair of eyeballs! *Lizzie*

How to take this dose

Begin by looking straight in front of you and finding an anchor point – something that doesn't move, that you can look directly at. Choose something that's level with your gaze. If you're inside, this might be a chair, a lamp or a painting on the wall. If you're outside, this might be a tree or a house.

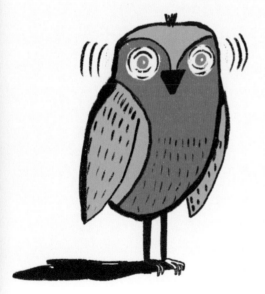

Focus your eyes on your anchor point. Once you've got that locked in, stretch your arms out in front of you and, while continuing to focus your vision on your anchor point, start wiggling your fingers way out in front of you.

Keep your gaze on your anchor while still wiggling your fingers. Slowly begin to move your arms apart from each other but continue to wiggle your fingers. Keep slowly moving your hands apart, stretching them wide, all the while keeping your eyes focused on your anchor. Keep spreading your arms out wide towards the sides of your body, until you just notice the wiggling fingers in your wide-angle vision, all the while continuing to maintain the anchor point in your gaze.

You'll likely lose focus on the details of the anchor point, but you are beginning to engage that wide peripheral vision that tends to perceive more movement. You can begin to take in 180 degrees of movement, and you'll see more of what is around you. As you see things and movements, you can zoom back in to your focused view, and then slip right back to Owl Eyes as desired. Try slowly turning your head from side to side, keeping your vision wide as you do so, and take in the breadth of the world where you are right at that moment.

Benefits

This technique can be a great way to help create a sense of expansion in your mind. It boosts our observation skills and can assist with widening our thinking and response to what is going on around us. It very quickly promotes the art of noticing, which can help ease us out of a busy mindset. It is a practice that builds curiosity and safekeeping.

The sensory experience of moving our arms, fingers and then holding a fixed gaze disrupts dysregulation in the nervous system, helping to calm the mind and return us to our Window of Tolerance (see page 121).

Relief

Clay Spheres

MEDIUM

Crafting & Making

TIME NEEDED

5–15 minutes

MATERIALS

- A decent handful of clay

Working with clay is an ancient practice that has been around for tens of thousands of years. This prescription is inspired by Korean artist Kimsooja, whose work, *Archive of Mind* (2017), we saw at the Art Gallery of New South Wales in 2023. In this participatory artwork, Kimsooja invites viewers to roll hunks of clay into balls and experience an immediate sense of calm. We have brought this practice to people in vulnerable states and witnessed how wonderfully grounding a sensory experience like this can be.

How to take this dose

You will need access to clay. A bag of natural clay can last indefinitely if covered. If you don't have the means or ability to get some, you can also make some. There are thousands of recipes on the internet for homemade playdough, the next best thing!

Grab a lump of clay with your hands and squeeze it, then roll it in your hands, around and around, to form a sphere.

You can take as long as you like to do this.

Make one to three spheres (more if you like) and place them in front of you. Notice how you feel as you sit in the quiet and calm space that you have created for yourself through this process.

Benefits

Research has shown that working with clay can have many benefits, acting as an immediate sensory meditation. The act of shaping and literally pressing earth with our hands can bring a symbolic sense of control and agency. The physical, sensual and mental experience of squishing it in our hands and pressing it with our palms promotes a sense of mindfulness and play.

As we shape and smooth and press and squash our clay, changing its shape in an instant, we're reminded of the imperfection and impermanence that surrounds us.

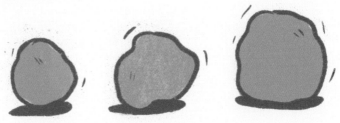

Relief

Write What You See

TIME NEEDED

5–10 minutes

MATERIALS

● A timer
● A piece of A4 paper
● A pen

We learnt this practice from working with award-winning young adult fiction author and writing teacher Helena Fox. She has led hundreds of people through short, playful creative writing practices at MakeShift that always leave people reporting that they feel more awake, alive, refreshed and calm.

How to take this dose

Find somewhere to sit or be comfy that gives you a view (through a window or doorway) of the outside. This provides a frame. If being able to see out through a window or doorway is hard, just choose a corner of the room or space to focus on.

Set a timer for 5 minutes. Get comfortable and plant your feet on the floor.

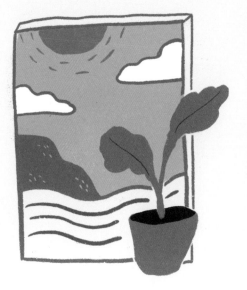

Start writing by just describing what you see. Try to use details. For example, 'I can see a brown terracotta pot plant. It's got dirt scraped on one side. A twisted, half-dying palm is growing out of it, about two metres high. The palm is flapping in the wind.' Continue to write and describe everything you can see, hear and smell. Don't edit, just write. Get it out. If you notice your focus wanders, that's okay, just bring yourself back. It's a lot like meditation!

When the timer goes off, put your pen down.

Take a moment to stretch and take a few deep breaths. Do a brief body scan. What do you notice in your body? What sensations are you experiencing?

Take a minute to read what you've written. Something within it might give you a jolt of inspiration to do something else. Maybe you want to keep writing. Maybe you don't. You can fold up the paper, or close your notebook, and never read it again!

Benefits

Writing can take us on a journey in our minds. We can imagine anything we like, and then write it down. It can also help us to release, play and care for ourselves in ways that talking can't. Sometimes seeing words on paper lands differently from actually saying them.

Writing by hand engages our sensory functions, which can help to regulate the nervous system. It slows us down, prompting us to choose our words more carefully. If we find ourselves stuck listening to the negative voices in our head, working to write in a loving way towards ourselves can foster self-compassion.

Creating a frame – through a window or door – and just writing out all that we see can offer a sense of release. Putting a boundary around what we write about can also bring a feeling of control. When everything feels huge and overwhelming, this practice can help bring things back to a small, contained window by connecting our sense of sight with our sense of touch.

Relief

Holding Hands

TIME NEEDED

5–10 minutes

MATERIALS

- A piece of A4 or A5 paper
- Something to make a mark with (a pencil, Sharpie, charcoal, texta, crayon, etc. – you'll need four different types)

This is something I used to do alongside my kids when they were little, and also asked them to do while I lay on the ground and they traced my hands – a moment to lie down! Our hands are things of wonder. They carry, push, pull, point, write, make, soothe, love. This simple drawing exercise, which has us slow down and trace a line, helps to engage the prefrontal cortex of the brain. Ensuring that the lines are parallel requires concentration, which moves us into the present, calming down the amygdala, the central HQ of our stress response system. Finding flow in the repetition can also let our mind wander towards the wonder of our hands – their unique shape, what they hold and the power and strength they give us. *Caitlin*

How to take this dose

❋ Trace your hands onto the paper.
❋ Find another three types of implements to make marks with (pencils, charcoal, markers); maybe they are different colours. Trace parallel lines around your hands, filling the page.
❋ As you make these lines, notice your breath. Slow down into the flowing movement of drawing the shape of your hand.

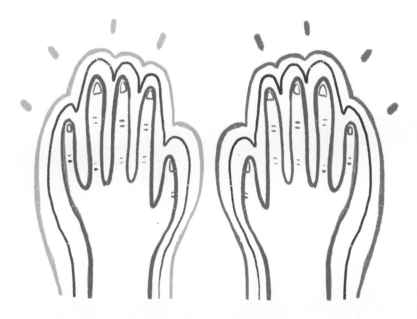

* Notice the length of each finger, the breadth of the palm – this body part that literally holds so many things for us.
* If you want to take it further, you can explore and play with any kind of pattern-making or drawing to fill in the hand, or even play with the space around the hand on the page. Circles, dots, faces, smaller hands, collage – whatever you like, there are no rules!

Benefits

Drawing without too much brain strain can work as a sensory meditation that gets us into that state of flow. We are being guided by a shape that brings movement to our marker on the page, and the sensory act of that helps to regulate our nervous system and bring us into the present moment.

Focusing on drawing a part of our body, one that we can sometimes take for granted, can help us connect with our body, and also bring some kindness towards ourselves, as we become thankful for those hands.

By making these hand shapes, and then filling them with anything we like, we can bring ourselves closer to a state of playfulness, of flow.

Relief

Humming

TIME NEEDED

1–2 minutes

MATERIALS

- Your voice

Sarah Ball is a trauma-sensitive and mental-health-focused yoga teacher, teacher trainer and mentor. She is a well-respected and authentic voice in our local community and has a beautiful ability of gifting wisdom without ego. During lunch with her one day, when we admitted to mutual admiration, we found a spark of collaboration in this sound-based practice, which is the heartbeat of Sarah's great work.

How to take this dose

When you feel ready, take a steady inhale. As you start to exhale, you might like to bring your lips together and ever so gently begin to make a humming sound. You can explore this sound all the way to the end of the exhalation, and then repeat as many times as you choose.

Perhaps you notice the sensation of your lips vibrating with the sound. Maybe you feel the sense of your belly moving as you breathe. As you hum, you can play with volume, and maybe even bring some spontaneous melody to the sound of your humming. Or you can use a more meditative, repetitive sound that allows you to unwind into the repetition. You choose.

Benefits

This activity is perfect for when you need to settle your system but need to stay where you are and so can't move around much. It's for when you're thinking more than feels helpful and you need to take a little pause but don't have long. It's for when you're not sure what to do to help yourself feel soothed.

When you hum, you invite the activation of the innate rest/digest response in your nervous system. This is likely (at least in part) because it's the opposite of how when we're under threat we breathe quickly to help fuel the fight/flight response. So when you breathe slowly on the exhale while humming or singing, you teach your nervous system that it's safe to unwind. The rhythmic nature of humming to the cycle of the breath can help to re-establish a sense of connection to natural rhythms, from which we can easily become disconnected amidst the frenetic pace of everyday life.

This exercise can be layered with other creative practices to support mindfulness. Best of all, because you always have your body with you, you can hum or play with your voice any time.

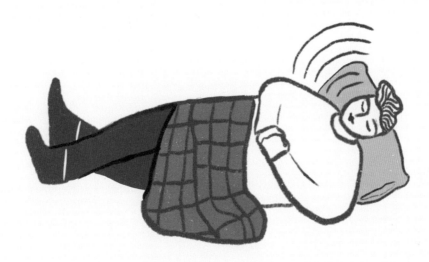

Relief

Toddler Tray

TIME NEEDED

5–10 minutes

MATERIALS

- A base plate or tray of some kind
- A drinking vessel
- 3–5 items of food that you find nourishing

This practice comes from our friend Nessie John. She is an environmental strategist, writer and design thinker. She is someone who is stacked full to the brim with ideas; in fact Nessie is the brains behind the name of our organisation, MakeShift. She designed this practice as a purposeful, creative act of self-care. It has room for her special blotchy mug, a water glass and snacks – sometimes a thermos. Her idea is that the slightly whimsical act of pulling this tray together offers both nutrition and kindness. 'I call it my Toddler Tray,' says Nessie, 'like how you might prep a lunchbox or pack an emergency banana for a kid in case of meltdown. We all melt down.'

How to take this dose

Choose your favourite plate, tray, chopping board or lunchbox as the 'base'. There can be something special in the ritual of using the same nice things each time. Then select your favourite cup, plate, fork or spoon. Perhaps even include a tea strainer.

Prepare the food. Choose nourishing snacks you can graze on, that you have on hand and that you enjoy. Make your tray look lovely and inviting; perhaps add a vase with a flower.

Go about your day with this plate on your desk as a reminder to slowly graze for energy, for both your body and your mind.

Benefits

This is a wonderful practice for when you're working at home alone and feeling jittery or alternatively a bit numb. Making a Toddler Tray can help to regulate your nervous system and bring about balance. It is also an adorable thing to prepare for someone. As Hippocrates said, 'Let food be thy medicine.'

Many of us experience complex feelings around food and our bodies. Sometimes we can struggle to identify biological signals of hunger and thirst, especially when we are busy or jittery. We can forget to eat, or we eat on the fly, in a hurry and without pausing other activities or resting hyperactive systems to prioritise digestion. For some of us, thoughts around food intake are preoccupying and stressful.

This practice can help to reduce overwhelm, and is a flexible, options-based style of offering ourselves nourishment, no matter what state we are in. Preparing food is also a creative process of consultation with the body. It is an act of profound care and demonstrates safety and resourcefulness to our entire internal system. Additionally, it can help wake up our nervous system, regulating us by following steps and doing repetitive actions like chopping, slicing, grating and even arranging items on a plate.

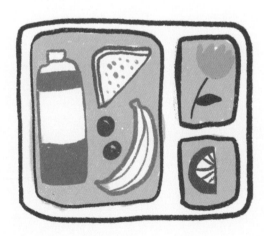

Relief

Six Directions

TIME NEEDED

1–5 minutes

MATERIALS

● A chair, towel, bed or yoga mat (basically something to sit, stand or kneel upon)

This practice was gifted to us to share by our friend, trauma-sensitive and mental-health-focused yoga teacher, Sarah Ball.

How to take this dose

In this practice, we explore the different ways the spine can move. You can explore this range of movements in a variety of positions, from sitting or standing to kneeling on the ground. Try to choose a place to find stillness that will allow for free movement of your spine.

Movement 1: Curls
✸ Inhale and press the front of your chest forward and draw your shoulders and hips back so your spine arcs forward.
✸ Exhale and invite your spine to draw backward so that your shoulders move in and down, and your hips curl inwards.
✸ Repeat this range of movement as many times as you wish.

Movement 2: Side to side

* Shift to the lateral movements, inviting your spine to move side to side, dropping your right shoulder down toward your right hip and perhaps lifting your left arm up and over to your right side on your exhalation.
* On your inhale, you can come back to a neutral spine, and then when you're ready to exhale, follow your breath by moving over to the left side, with your right arm reaching up and over to the left side of your body.
* Repeat as many times as feels good for you.

Movement 3: Twist

* Twist your spine by turning from side to side. There are many ways to twist, which can include rapid micro-twists or longer holds.
* You can play with swinging your arms and twisting in (gentle!) ways in both directions, or pausing and breathing in one place, as you choose.

Benefits

This is a great practice for when you're feeling agitated or stuck, and need some help shifting gears. When we move mindfully, we help revitalise our body in a very gentle way by increasing circulation and respiration. Gentle movements can also provide a nice counterbalance to the postural locks we can find ourselves in, especially if we work sitting down a lot. Reconnecting with our body can make spontaneous movement and play possible. It also gives us a structure to lean into if we're experiencing decision fatigue.

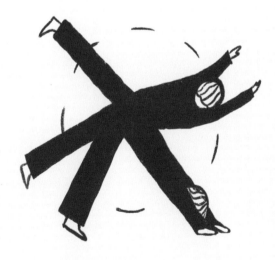

Relief

Pause for a Poem

TIME NEEDED

1–3 minutes

MATERIALS

- Your eyes

This poem was written by our friend Kirli Saunders (OAM). Kirli is a proud Gunai woman and award-winning international writer of poetry, plays and picture books. She is a teacher, cultural consultant and artist. In 2020, Kirli was named the NSW Aboriginal Woman of the Year. Kirli works with MakeShift as a creative facilitator, and this poem is one that we have been sharing with participants as part of our programs for years. It speaks to the need for self-care but, as Kirli notes, it is really about the idea that carving out time to look after ourselves has positive impacts that ripple out into the community, allowing us to show up for our friends and family.

How to take this dose

Take a moment to get comfy. You can even put the kettle on and make yourself a cup of tea. Then read this poem.

Self Care
from *Kindred*
(Magabala Books, 2019)

step off the grid
write instead

pour tea

find melodies
that mimic heartbeats

s t r e t c h
and breathe

contemplate
why honeysuckle always
climbs the tree clockwise

if it is the sun
who chases
the moon
or vice versa

why we look
at plant skeletons
and see
homes

could we see
that home
in our own
bones?

swim, sweat
or cry

eat something green

rinse
and repeat

rinse
and repeat

Benefits

Reading poetry brings us into the present, helping us to slow down and shift our perspective.

It can also offer an emotional boost and provide us with a glimmer of beauty, joy and wonder.

Recharge

Bilateral Drawing

MEDIUM

Mark Making

TIME NEEDED

Start with 2 minutes

MATERIALS

- **A piece of A4 paper**
- **Two drawing implements (pens, pencils, textas, Sharpies, etc.)**

We love this simple drawing practice. Bilateral stimulation is an incredibly soothing exercise for our nervous system. It works to create electrical activity in different parts of the brain, encouraging better communication between the right and left sides. Clinical psychologists often engage with this concept through treatments such as EMDR therapy (Eye Movement Desensitisation and Reprocessing), which uses bilateral eye stimulation to rewire neural pathways.

How to take this dose

Bilateral literally means 'both sides', so this exercise uses your left and right hand to create simultaneous marks on paper that mirror one another.

Get your paper and do this either sitting or standing – whatever feels right.

Place a pen (or whichever drawing implement you desire) in each hand and begin doodling patterns on the page with both hands.

The idea isn't to create an image, but to make mirrored patterns of swirls, circles or anything you like. Feel free to change colours throughout.

Continue until the page is filled.

Optional extras:
* Listen to music while you draw bilaterally.
* Experiment with different sizes of paper; larger pieces allow you to make bigger patterns.

Benefits

Bilateral drawing can connect us to our bodies and our rhythms. It warms up our brains for left and right thinking, firing up our creative muscle.

Using our non-dominant hand helps to bring us into a state of mindful flow, as our brain is focused on doing something new in an unusual way. This makes it harder to stay locked in thinking about yesterday or tomorrow and brings us into the present instead.

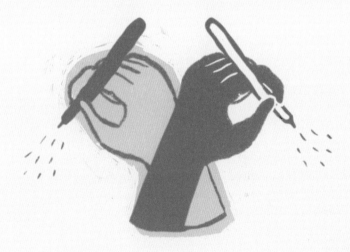

Recharge

Cold-water Swimming

TIME NEEDED

1–10 minutes

MATERIALS

- A body of water (you can use a bath with ice, too)
- Swimming gear
- Warm clothing (for afterwards)
- A thermos of tea (optional)

There are ten sea pools within a 10-minute drive from where I live on Dharawal land. I feel gratitude to these pools for getting me through life's tricky moments, including a pandemic. They are also where my kids learnt to swim. Plunging into an ocean pool snaps me back into myself almost instantly; it is sometimes the only place I can turn off all the tabs in my brain. I've been swimming regularly for five years, long enough to have become somewhat evangelical about it. **Lizzie**

How to take this dose

'You never regret a swim,' says every regular swimmer, ever. This is a prescription that is being very relaxed about the definition of creativity. The creative part is all in the mindset and how we approach such things.

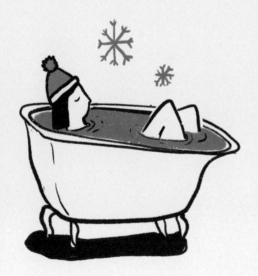

Remember, there is a difference between self-soothing – doing something that makes us feel good and brings immediate relief – and self-care – an act that can be harder to start, but shifts us through an experience, making us feel something different afterwards.

So prepare yourself. Before you enter the cold water, quieten the voice yelling at you to stop being ridiculous. Trust yourself that it will be worth it. Remind yourself that this is seconds, maybe minutes of your life, and it is medicine worth taking. You've got this!

Jump, dive, or inch, depending on your individual style, into the water. Feel it surround you, the sharp sting on your skin, the fright of cold on your head and ears. Take a moment to feel it all. Try to go under at least three times. Jump up and down. Shout and exclaim! Whoop and holler! It can help. This is you in your most basic, animal form.

If possible, try to stay in the water for at least 3 minutes, letting your body adapt and settle as it understands the sudden new space you are in. Feel weightless, float. Then retreat to your towel, your jumper, your thermos of tea. Notice the feeling – no doubt different to just minutes ago. Notice the sense of freshness, of a cleaning-out of your brain, of an aliveness, a high. Hold onto that. Take it with you.

If you can't access cold water, or even water to swim in, putting ice cubes in a bowl with water and then putting your hands in it can take you through a similar sensory experience.

Benefits

Jumping in cold water improves circulation. It also increases our heart rate, making it a fast-tracked form of physical exercise. Some studies suggest that cold-water submersion burns more calories per minute than walking, gym workouts or boxing.

Research into the benefits of cold-water swimming has found that the practice gives us an opportunity to teach our body to adapt to stress. The initial shock of cold to the body thrusts us into a fight/flight response, as the body perceives pain in the form of cold and the amygdala floods our nervous system with adrenaline and endorphins to cope, then prompts that feeling of elation or 'post-swim high'. By giving ourselves a chance to experience a nervous system shock, and then learn to adapt to it, we can be more resilient when we face stress in our lives.

That moment before we jump in the cold water is like many moments we face in life. It can be hard to begin, especially when we know it would be way more comfortable to grab our woolly jumper and a hot cup of tea. But if we take the plunge and learn to manage the cold, we know it will be good for us and make us feel better in the long run.

Recharge

Paint Blobbing

TIME NEEDED

1–5 minutes

MATERIALS

- A piece of A4 paper
- A paintbrush
- Watercolour or acrylic paints
- A glass of water

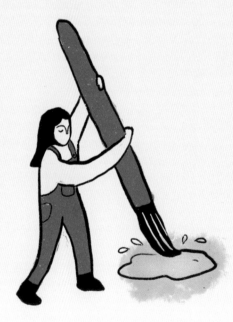

Kiara Mucci, the illustrator of this book, brought paint blobbing to our programs as a grounding practice. She says that if you don't know where to start with painting, watercolour can be a good entry point as it is so forgiving.

How to take this dose

✳ Start with your brush in a glass of clear water, then make big water blobs on your piece of paper. See if you can fit six blobs on the page.

✳ Dip the brush into some colour, then dab the brush into the water on the page and watch it fill.

✳ Move the colour around, noticing the sensation of pushing colour through the water, the way it trails, bends and blends.

✳ Keep on blobbing! Be bold – try out different-sized blobs.

Benefits

The sensory input of water, paint and paintbrushes can help to soothe an activated nervous system. Feeling the sensation of pushing water and paint around the paper can promote mindfulness and bring us into that state of playful flow.

Recharge

Making Sounds

MEDIUM

Music
& Sound

TIME NEEDED

Start with 2 minutes

MATERIALS

● **Your voice and body**

Our nervous system can be altered by making sounds, as it quickly activates the vagus nerve, which is like a conductor for our nervous system. Using our vocal cords to create sounds is very effective in relieving stress, anxiety and overwhelm.

How to take this dose

✱ Stand with your feet firmly on the ground. Place one hand on your belly and one on your chest. Start with a strong, loud, 'HA.' Repeat, noticing and feeling where that sound vibrates in your body. Turn it into a long 'HMMMM.' Repeat, again feeling the vibrations. Now, try 'HOOOOO.'

✱ Finish with a big breath and a long, loud sigh – 'Haaaaaaah.' Repeat this whole cycle, using MA, MMMM and MOOOO. Enjoy!

Benefits

This technique is used by singers and music therapists to unlock and loosen vocal cords, release tension and create energy in the voice. Trauma therapists also use humming, singing and chanting to stimulate the vagus nerve (see page 116), which helps us relax faster after experiencing stress.

Recharge

Body Weather Mapping

MEDIUM

Movement

TIME NEEDED

10–20 minutes

MATERIALS

● **Your body**
● **A comfortable place to lie or sit**

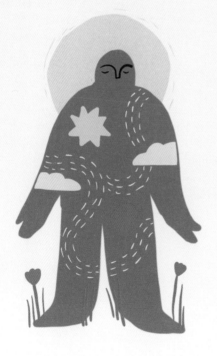

This practice was gifted to us by Sarah Ball, who trains practitioners in trauma-sensitive yoga and movement.

How to take this dose

This is a practice used in yoga and meditation and can also be called S-BSET, which is an acronym for sound, breath, sensation, emotion, thought.

Lie or sit as comfortably as you can, in whatever position works for you. Can you do a final adjustment to make yourself 10 per cent more comfortable?

Sound
Bring your awareness to the sounds around you – sounds outside the room; sounds inside the room.

Breath
Start to notice that your body is breathing by itself. Do you notice any movement in your mouth or nostrils, your neck, throat, shoulders, chest or belly? This is not about changing your breath, or labelling it as good or bad – just notice it.

Sensation

Begin to widen the scope of your awareness, from your breath to other sensations in your body. You might notice the sensation of your body in contact with the surface beneath you. Maybe you feel sensations of clothing on skin, and of the shape of your body in whatever position you're in. You might notice sensations of temperature on your skin.

Emotion

Gently redirect your awareness from physical sensations towards the landscape of your emotional experience. Are there any words that might describe how you are feeling right now? If not, that's okay. Can you notice where you feel a sense of emotion in your body? How does your body feel when you invite emotions to be present? If this concept of emotions in the body feels confusing, simply notice that confusion arising. Be open to curiosity, offering gentleness towards any emotions that may be present.

Thought

Turn the spotlight of your awareness towards your mind now. As you observe your mind thinking, you might notice that, just as the body breathes itself, the mind also 'thinks itself' without any particular effort on your part. You might notice that the mind is constantly narrating your experience, whether you're paying attention to it or not. The mind chatters to itself about all sorts of things, forming opinions, ideas, judgements and preferences. Can you also notice that a part of yourself is able to stand aside and watch this chatter?

After cycling through these mindful observations, return to just lying and breathing, and not focusing on anything much at all. When you feel ready, you can open your eyes and sit up.

Benefits

Tuning in to the unconscious processes of our bodies can also help us tune in to more conscious ones. By learning to notice sounds, the breath, sensations, thoughts and emotions, we bring ourselves into the present, helping to ground and regulate us into our Window of Tolerance (see page 121).

By practising this mindfully and without judgement, we cultivate self-compassion and curiosity, which are key foundations of applying creative first aid.

Recharge

Loud, Quiet, Loud

MEDIUM

Nature & Adventure

TIME NEEDED

Start with 10 minutes

MATERIALS

● **A cushion (optional)**

The world is noisy. We can be so busy in our days and life that we don't even notice the hundreds of noises – pings of a phone, people talking, the hum of appliances, radios. Sometimes, when we are in a heightened, anxious state, all those noises get even louder and more abrasive. Or when we are disconnected and frozen, we are completely tuned out to any noise at all.

For anyone who is sensitive to noise – but who also loves many, many types of sounds – this is a lovely way to quieten the sharp throng of noise, and instead tune in to the sounds (even the most delicate, quiet ones) of nature.

How to take this dose

This practice is about exploring the difference between noise and sound.

Noise can be jarring, a cacophony that assaults our senses and contributes to feeling overwhelm, whereas the right dose of sound can calm our nervous system, help us focus and promote relaxation.

Starting with sounds out there in the world, this prescription is an exploration of sound through your connection with nature.

Find a spot to sit somewhere outside that's private and comfortable, perhaps on a cushion. (Preferably you can find a spot in nature in a park or in your garden.) The idea is to use your ears like binoculars, homing in on just one or two sounds.

Start by just sitting and listening. Close your eyes if it's helpful.

See if you can locate and identify all the different sounds you can hear – the tiny crackling of leaves, birds chirping, the hum of traffic, people talking, phones beeping.

After a few minutes, latch onto one sound. Perhaps it is a single bird call, or the rustle of a particular tree branch. Try to follow that one sound so closely that all the other sounds fade away.

Pay close attention to that sound. Is it changing? What are its qualities? These can be useful reflections, but it might also feel nice just to let that sound wash over and through you, without examining it too much.

Benefits

Sound is a powerful regulating experience for humans. The first sound we hear is the heartbeat of our mother in the womb. When we tune in to our auditory system, our brains light up more than when we use any other sense.

By using our 'ears as binoculars' we can train them to tune in to sounds that provide pleasure, interest, wonder or delight. We can build this practice, which enables us to feel more in control in times when the noise of the world can feel like an assault on our senses.

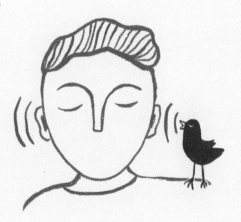

Recharge

Hirameki

TIME NEEDED

10–15 minutes

MATERIALS

- A piece of A3 or A2 paper (the bigger the better)
- Ink or watercolour paints
- A paintbrush, or a cloth to dab blobs of paint or ink with
- Something to draw with (a pen, Sharpie, texta, etc.)

Hirameki means 'brainwave' or 'flash of inspiration' and is a Japanese art form. Giving ourselves the opportunity to get that 'flash' can be such a fun spark of delight and surprise. This practice was shared with us by comic illustrator and MakeShift drawing facilitator Marcelo Baez when we first began developing the methodology for this book. We had gathered a group of eight creative facilitators with whom we intended to work to test out these activities. Marcelo arrived with a huge sheet of paper covered in coloured blobs. We laid it out in the middle of our office desk and stood around it in a circle. 'Draw what you see,' he said and, without overthinking it, we each drew creatures, characters, small scenes and scenarios using the blobs on the page. It was great fun, offering us an instant portal into our creativity, and the end result looked pretty amazing, too!

How to take this dose

Begin with a clean, blank piece of paper.

Using your ink or watercolour paints, pick up your paintbrush and create splashes and blobs of colour all over the paper. Allow them to dry.

Walk away from the paper for a few minutes and take a look at the blobs with fresh eyes. Grab a pen or texta. Look for shapes that spark inspiration and use them to create something else entirely – imaginative creatures, funny faces, plants, animals, whatever brainwave strikes you. You can add arms, legs, eyes or even wings and a tail! You should end up with an entire menagerie of original drawings.

Benefits

This activity is great at bringing us into the present and firing up our imagination by giving us a little puzzle to solve, i.e. finding things to draw out of the blobs of paint. This practice is a great way to kickstart creativity when you don't know where to begin. It's a playful way to get curious, too.

The sensory act of painting and drawing can also help to calm our nervous system, reducing levels of cortisol (the hormone that makes us feel stressed) and bringing us into our Window of Tolerance (see page 121).

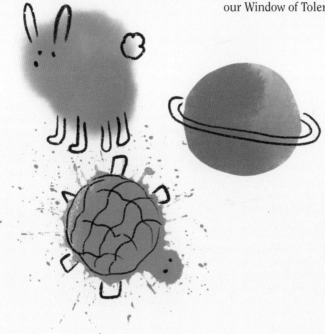

Recharge

Walking Bingo

TIME NEEDED

20 minutes or more

MATERIALS

- Walking bingo card
  (just take a photo of
  the illustration here,
  or make your own)
- If you're making
  your own, you will
  need a piece of paper
  or card, and a pen or
  pencil

Illustrator and MakeShift creative facilitator
Kiara Mucci designed this practice during
the coronavirus pandemic. It helped a lot of
people and families stay connected to each
other and to nature while in lockdown. This
practice can be done in a city setting, in the
country, in the 'burbs – wherever!

'Coddiwomple' is an English slang word
that means 'to travel in a purposeful manner
towards a vague destination'. The vagueness
is an opportunity for mind-wandering
and daydreaming, two critical ingredients
that enable us to generate ideas and
solve problems.

How to take this dose

* Using your bingo card as a guide, go for
  a walk around your neighbourhood, taking
  note of what to look for and crossing off
  items as you go along.
* You don't have to find everything on the
  card in one walk; you can do it over a few
  days or a week.

Benefits

Taking a walk outside is one of the simplest and most effective ways to calm our nervous system. Walking is a bilateral movement (i.e. it requires the use of the left and right sides of the body at the same time) and can help to disrupt dysregulated signals in our bodies, amping up our endorphins.

This activity also invokes curiosity, play and wonder. By having a task to focus on as we walk, we're not left to ruminate on our thoughts and worries. Walking Bingo offers a unique way to get some fresh air and explore your neighbourhood.

a succulent	something older than you	water	something broken
a feather	something edible	3 kinds of birds	a double-number mailbox 3 3
something handmade	peeling paint	a bit of graffiti	something spikey
a wave to a neighbour	a rock shaped like an animal	a colourful leaf	something younger than you

Recharge

Foliage Forage

Nature & Adventure

TIME NEEDED

10–30 minutes

MATERIALS

- Access to plants and flowers (i.e. your neighbourhood, a local park, etc.)
- A jar or vase of water

Karen Yello has been a part of our team since the very beginning. We have run hundreds of workshops and events that also come with many planning meetings. There hasn't been a single time that Karen hasn't turned up to these meetings or workshops without a bunch of foraged foliage in her hands. She constantly reminds us that snatching a flower or two brings joy!

How to take this dose

This prescription will depend a lot on where you live, and what's around you when you walk out the door.

Exploring your neighbourhood or local parklands can be a great and easy way to have a little adventure in flora foraging. If walking any real distance is tricky, you could stick to your own backyard, if you have one.

As you get out on your walk, look for leaves, branches and flowers that can be collected or picked. Perhaps they are on the nature strip. Sometimes there are amazing flowers growing in large supermarket carparks. (Remember to ask permission before taking foliage from someone's property.)

Bring what you collect home (it doesn't have to be florist-standard!). Find a jar or vase and spend a little time arranging the flora into a pleasing posy or bouquet. This little bunch of nature's delight can now exist in your space for a time.

Benefits

Not only can foraging for local plants and flowers help us to create a feeling of connection and belonging with our neighbourhood, it can also be fun and exploratory!

The zing of joy that comes with creating a bouquet of foliage gives us a hit of dopamine, the chemical in our brains that brings warm fuzzy feelings.

This practice also helps remind us that we have the power to bring beauty and delight into the space we are in. Having indoor plants and foliage has also been proven to help lower blood pressure, heart rate and stress hormones, regulating our nervous system more broadly. We can also engage our senses by touching each stem, flower, twig and leaf, and breathing in their earthy, perfumed aromas.

Recharge

Your Perfect Day

TIME NEEDED

15 minutes

MATERIALS

- A piece of A4 paper
- A pen or pencil
- Coloured pencils
  or markers

Annie Werner, whom we met in Chapter 1, sat us down one day and asked us, 'What would your perfect day look like?' We each grabbed a piece of paper and she took us through this activity. Her intention was to have us experience even just a little bit of our perfect day on a regular basis.

How to take this dose

This exercise is best done with a warm pot of tea and your shoes off. Having your favourite music playing in the background can be nice.

Write or draw the elements that would make up a perfect day for you. Where would you be? What would you be doing? Are you alone or with people? Are you somewhere familiar or foreign? What's the weather like? What sounds can you hear? What can you taste?

Don't overthink this too much, just write down what comes to mind when you imagine a perfect day.

Pin this up on your wall or fold it and put it in your drawer. See if over the next fortnight you can carve out time to enact this kind of day you have dreamed up, even if it's only a small part of it.

Benefits

This activity works as a form of radical self-care and it can help to increase feelings of self-worth. It acts as a refill of your reserves.

The process of engaging our imagination and writing about our hopes and dreams exercises our storytelling muscle. This can disrupt anxious, busy brains and tired bodies. It gives us a moment to envisage a possible day in the future, helping us to zoom out on this current moment and see the bigger picture.

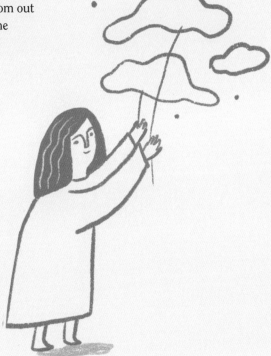

Recharge

Making Pompoms

TIME NEEDED

10 minutes

MATERIALS

- Yarn
- A pair of scissors

This practice was taught to us by a participant at a large-scale event we held in the forest on Dharawal land, where 100 adults came together to retreat from the busyness of life and work. With the sun streaming, we sat on the grass and made over 300 pompoms, and the result was a connected group of calm and happy people, as well as coloured pompoms everywhere.

How to take this dose

This practice is portable – you can do it anywhere and any time you need to keep your hands busy. It's addictive and simple!

✳ Take the end of a ball of yarn and start winding it around four of your fingers, securing the end with your thumb.

✳ Keep winding the yarn around your four fingers at least 30 times, or as many times as you like – the more you wind, the thicker the pompom will be. Make sure you don't wind too tightly!

✳ Snip the end of the yarn to release it from the ball.

✳ Carefully slide the bundle of yarn off your fingers so that it stays together.

* Cut a piece of yarn about 10–15 cm
  (4–6 inches) long. Wrap the yarn around
  the middle of your bundle of yarn, as if
  you're tying a ribbon on a gift, and tie
  it once on the top of your bundle, then
  once on the bottom of your bundle.
  You should now have a tightly knotted
  bundle of yarn loops.
* Carefully cut through the loops of the
  bundle, all the way around.
* To finish, you can trim your pompom to
  neaten up the ends. You can either trim
  the longest piece of yarn that remains, or
  use it to tie your pompom to something.
* Repeat as many times as you like to
  make several pompoms. You can hang a
  bunch of coloured pompoms anywhere
  to bring a small moment of joy – off
  your car's rear-view mirror, on your
  Christmas tree, in a kid's bedroom
  or beside the kitchen window!

Benefits

Keeping our hands busy helps promote a
calm mind. The repetitive nature of this
kind of practice has been proven to release
serotonin, the key hormone in stabilising
our mood, feelings of wellbeing, and
happiness – it's a natural antidepressant!

The repetitive movement also acts as a
meditation, bringing a sense of mindfulness
and propelling us into that zone of flow,
calming our mind and body.

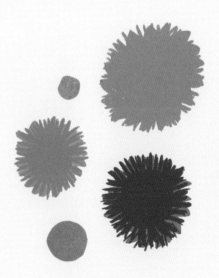

Recharge

Visual Poetry

MEDIUM

Writing &
Mark Making

TIME NEEDED

10–20 minutes

MATERIALS

- Several pieces of A4
  or A3 paper
- A pen
- Some coloured
  pencils or markers

Proud Gunai woman, award-winning writer
and visual artist, consultant, speaker and
facilitator Kirli Saunders (OAM) shared
this practice at a workshop we ran together
at the Sydney Opera House, in the Centre
for Creativity. Kirli's practice brings together
multiple forms, including writing, poetry
reading, drawing, painting, meditation
and nature connection. This prescription
invites you to explore both writing and
mark making in a meditative, mindful way.
You don't need to have any experience at
writing poetry, or drawing for that matter!

How to take this dose

Begin by getting comfortable. Tune in to
your breathing and feel your feet grounded
on the floor, on Country, wherever that
may be.

Let your mind take you to a place that feels
alive, safe, and full of life and possibility,
preferably outside, on Country. Maybe it's
a garden, a valley or a forest. Maybe it's a
beach, a cave or a riverbank.

Without thinking too hard, write down
five words or statements that define, explain
or transmit the feeling of this place for you.

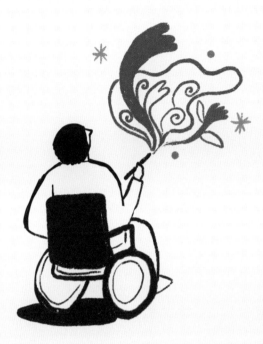

They could be words about the colours, textures and sensations of this place or they could describe how this place makes you feel.

Take a new piece of paper and, using a coloured pencil or marker, write a poem that expands on one of those phrases or words you've written. You might like to set this poem against a pattern, or background, or image that you draw. Play around with writing words visually, e.g. writing the word 'wavy' in a curve or making the word 'big' larger than the others.

You've made a visual poem!

Benefits

Exploring our imagination through words is an act of release and play. Writing poetry about a specific place can invoke a range of feelings about home, safety and even the wonder of being truly alive.

Becoming absorbed in creating a visual picture of these words through mark making can help to slow down fast breathing, busy brains, and a sense of overwhelm.

The sensory acts of both writing and drawing help to regulate our nervous system. It can bring us closer to that mindful state of flow and play. Invoking and remembering places of beauty and nature that we have been to can take us outside a stressful day, or our current worries.

Recharge

Paper Portrait

MEDIUM

Crafting
& Making

Angie Cass is an analogue and digital collage artist and a regular MakeShift facilitator. Her process is to gather and group cut-outs and scraps of paper together and hunt for patterns, themes and colours. We have worked with Angie to bring stop-motion animation workshops to people from across Australia, absorbing her knowledge about the creative process through the craft of collage.

How to take this dose

This activity will result in a creation of your own image in a playful, fun way.

Don't worry too much about what the end result might look like. It's more important to open your imagination and explore the process of making a portrait of yourself, a friend or even a pet using only paper, glue and scissors.

Start by gathering your materials. When you have all the paper scraps you think you will need, play with them to make shapes and group colours together. Take note of any patterns that emerge as you go.

Now it's time to make a face! You might like to choose a colour for the face and cut out the shape. Then use the scraps to cut out some eyes, a nose, eyebrows, lips, ears and hair. Do you need to cut out a pair of glasses? Perhaps some earrings? A beard or even a moustache?

Arrange all the elements of your portrait on the piece of card, making a face.

When you are happy with the result, glue everything down onto the card.

Rather than having to draw or paint someone or something, making a collage just involves cutting and arranging paper in a unique way. It's a really low-stakes way to get creative and play.

The sensory experience of cutting, gluing and arranging can bring us into that mindful flow state. Creating a portrait of ourselves helps to promote self-compassion, as we think of ourselves in a new and different way.

Benefits

Angie describes collaging as a democratic craft because it doesn't require any experience, or particular skills besides being able to use scissors.

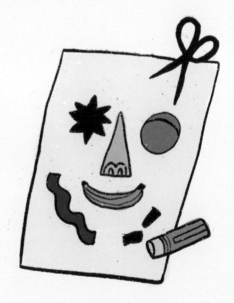

Recharge

Glimmer Hunting

MEDIUM

Nature &
Adventure

TIME NEEDED

5–10 minutes

MATERIALS

- A notebook
- A pen or pencil

We first thought about this idea as a practice after a conversation we had with friend and award-winning author Helena Fox. We were sitting by the sea, catching up on life and work, and then we began to talk about clouds. Helena described them as anchors that helped her get through tricky days. 'I hunt them out, watch them float by, look for shapes and creatures in them. Their constant shifting helps my mind shift,' she told us. This concept came up again when we went to a talk by author Heather Rose. She spoke of watching clouds pass by as a conscious act of joy and a way to manage the physical and mental pain she was in from an autoimmune disease. Glimmer hunting has since become a firm fixture in our programs and has proven to be an accessible way for people to grow their curiosity and promote joy. It refers to the concept of glimmers that we talked about on page 91. Glimmers are tiny moments, things and happenings that are a spark of soft, warm goodness.

How to take this dose

You can practise this activity anywhere – in an office, on a bus, at a train station – but it is best done outside if you can.

This is an observational practice; it's about taking time to look around you and then looking a little longer and a little deeper. It can take as long as ten minutes for something to reveal itself, but there will always be a small glimmer waiting to be harvested.

Move away from wherever you are and go to a space nearby. Notice what you see, what you hear, how you feel. Look left, then right; look up, down and all around. Then linger somewhere and just watch what is happening. What can you see? It might be as subtle as the flicker of a shadow moving past you.

If you see something that catches your eye, that makes you pay attention, pause there and notice it. You might have just collected a glimmer. Glimmers are a little beginning that can lead to joy.

Write down what you found in your notebook. Over time, if you practise this activity again and again, you'll build a list of glimmers that you can return to when you need them. Or just enjoy your glimmer and move on, knowing that such moments can be fleeting.

Benefits

This activity is a wonderful exercise for tuning in and noticing the good stuff – the joy, the beauty and the sparks that are happening around us. Sitting at the opposite end of the spectrum to triggers, glimmers (a concept conceived by trauma clinician and social worker Deb Dana), offer the opportunity to develop a practice of receiving and recognising joy.

Glimmer hunting builds curiosity. It helps us slow down and primes our nervous system to receive cues of delight, connection and safety.

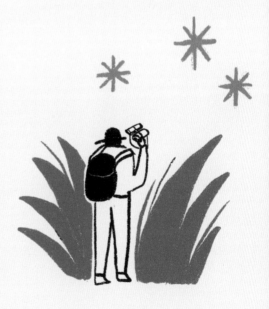

Recharge

Cut and Paste

MEDIUM

Crafting
& Making

TIME NEEDED

10–20 minutes

MATERIALS

- A piece of A4 paper
- Collaging materials, (wrapping paper, magazines, old cards, postcards, atlases, street maps, sheet music, etc.)
- A pair of scissors
- A glue stick

Angie Cass, collage artist and creative facilitator at MakeShift, shared this practice, and her passion for collage, through our programs and courses together. Collage can be a really simple-to-start creative practice, and you can create some beautiful, powerful imagery, too.

How to take this dose

✸ Take your collection of collaging materials and start cutting out things that catch your eye – there are no rules here.

✸ Arrange and glue your cut-outs on the sheet of paper. Perhaps a theme emerges, and you are creating a picture that is telling a story. Or maybe it's a nonsensical arrangement of things stuck on a page!

Benefits

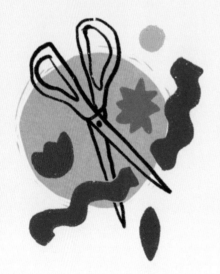

When we use scissors for collaging, we regulate our nervous system. By giving our brains lots to do – like concentrating on where we are cutting – we disrupt our busy, worried thoughts. Additionally, the sensory experience of feeling paper in our hands and moving it around helps to wake us up out of that foggy, exhausted freeze state. Creating something new out of scraps can bring a sense of accomplishment and purpose.

Recharge

Shadow Drawing

MEDIUM

Mark Making

We learnt this practice from artist and illustrator Kiara Mucci, who has also created all the illustrations in this book. Kiara has collaborated with us on our ReMind program and is also a member of the MakeShift team. Her life and work are deeply connected to nature, and she is always finding moments of inspiration through flowers, trees and the sea.

How to take this dose

✻ Take three big breaths, in and out. Notice any tension in different parts of your body.
✻ Sit comfortably, with the paper in front of you. Arrange a branch or twig in a way that it casts shadow across your paper.
✻ Trace around the shadow, taking care to capture the shape.
✻ If you feel compelled, you can embellish this shape with colour, shading or pattern.

Benefits

By slowing down and making repeat patterns, we engage the prefrontal cortex of the brain. We also get to practise drawing in a low-stakes way, tracing the shadow of something that already exists. This helps bring us into the present, and it connects us to living things in nature and objects, which also helps to lower our stress hormones.

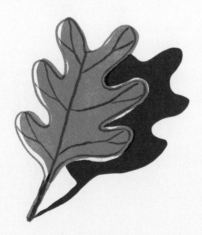

Recharge

Tiny and Giant, All at Once

MEDIUM

Nature & Adventure

TIME NEEDED

20 minutes

MATERIALS

- Yourself

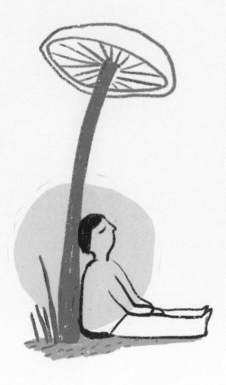

I read a book some years ago called *The Reality Bubble: Blind spots, hidden truths, and the dangerous illusions that shape our world* by Ziya Tong. It's mostly about how little humans actually see of the world we live in, such as how our food is made or where our waste goes. But the really interesting part for me was about how much happens on a tiny scale that humans are blind to. It talked about how most of actual life on earth is at this scale – tiny bugs, insects, organisms. We can start to see this on a forest floor. The book also talked about the vast and gigantic nature of other things, so large that we also don't see them.

I now reflect on this every time I'm in a forest, or near mountains. The scale of things brings a sense of perspective I find really comforting. I'm a tiny speck on the scale of the universe, and a giant that could crush a whole ant world under my feet if I'm not paying attention! *Caitlin*

How to take this dose

Take yourself to a tree-filled space. It could be a park, a garden, a forest or bushland. Turn your phone to silent and pause any notifications.

Start by inspecting the ground. What is the teeniest thing you can see that is alive? An ant? Moss? A fungus? Get right down into the world of that tiny thing. Imagine how giant we must seem to that ant, fungus or moss. How large we must loom to them. They are busy in their world, in that scale, hidden in the dead tree logs and under rocks and in little burrows and holes in the soil.

Stretch up from the ground and turn your attention upwards. Take in the height of tall, towering trees or large, epic rock faces. Look up at the sky, seeing it stretch into space. Notice the clouds or even the moon, or stars if they are beginning to appear. Remind yourself of how teeny-tiny you are at this scale. How, from way up there, your steps are like those tiny ant steps you were just watching at your feet.

Benefits

Staring at a screen for too long can be bad for our eyes. But research shows that lifting our head and looking out to a horizon every so often can help. Similarly, we can find some sense of perspective in being reminded that we are both tiny and giant all at once.

While we can feel like a small, insignificant speck in the world, this practice can bring a sense of how much influence we can have in a natural space on the billions of living organisms lying at our feet, hoping we don't step on them!

Likewise, being reminded that we are a tiny living thing on this giant planet, in an even more enormous solar system, can release us from being weighed down by too many worries and busy jobs. It can be a powerful reminder of the vastness of our universe, and our place in it. While this can be hard to conceptualise, there is some strange comfort in remembering that our lifetimes come and go, with all of the detail in them, and this helps us to remember what really matters.

Recharge

Brain Dance

TIME NEEDED

10 minutes

MATERIALS

- **Your body**

This practice was taught to us by choreographer, artist, director and performer Emma Saunders. We have used this dance many times with groups of people as a body/brain movement tool that assists with emotional regulation and social connection. Originally developed by renowned dancer, educator and author Anne Green Gilbert, the Brain Dance was adapted by Emma for her work with us, using movement to bring together creativity and mental health.

How to take this dose

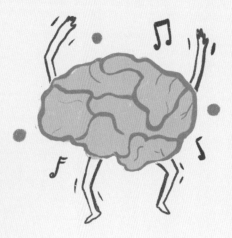

The Brain Dance can be done standing, lying down, or seated on the floor or on a chair. This prescription is a series of movements that use and interact with different elements and parts of our body. Choose a few, or do them all!

Breath: Exhale through the mouth gently, then inhale through the nose. Do this four to six times.

Touch: Firmly squeeze your arms with your hands, then squeeze your legs, your torso, back and head. Next, lightly tap your whole body using the tips of your fingers, then use your arms to hug your whole body. Finally, smoothly brush your whole body with your palms.

Core: Curl your body, including your arms and legs, inwards. Then stretch outwards, like a starfish.

Head to tail: With your knees slightly bent, gently bend, twist and stretch your spine from head to tail. Circle and swing your head and your hips. Any gentle movement that works to loosen the spine will work here.

Upper to lower: With the lower half of your body grounded and stable, and knees slightly bent, swing, bend, stretch and rotate the upper body in all directions and at different speeds. Then, ground the upper half of your body and dance with your lower half (feet, legs, hips).

Body side: Bend, twist, stretch and shake the left side of your body while keeping the right side stable. Then swap and do the other side. Next, like a lizard crawling up a wall, move your right and left sides by reaching your left arm and knee up, then your right arm and knee up.

Cross-lateral: Touch your right knee to your left elbow, then swap sides. Next, touch your left hand to your right foot, then swap sides. Repeat.

Balance: Twirl around in circles several times and then try balancing on one foot, a movement that takes you off balance and makes you slightly dizzy (slight dizziness followed by stabilisation stimulates and strengthens the balance system).

Benefits

This series of movements or 'dances' is designed to activate and engage our entire brain. It's an incredibly powerful somatic practice of movement.

The Brain Dance also helps to release stress and physical tension from the body, regulating our sensory system and grounding our central nervous system. Additionally, finding balance and using crossing movements can help to develop emotional stability and balance the body and nervous system, connecting the right and left brain and helping us feel present and in that ventral vagal state.

Recharge

Making a Plant Your Friend

MEDIUM

Nature & Adventure

TIME NEEDED

30 minutes, then
1 minute every day

MATERIALS

- A house plant (maybe a seedling, or one that's fully grown – it's up to you)
- A pot
- Some potting mix
- Spray bottle (optional)

Narelle Happ is a garden designer and horticulturist who specialises in native gardens and permaculture design. She has worked with us since the very beginning of our organisation, which means that over the past ten years we have learnt a lot about plants! Together we have worked with refugees in a community garden, brought bush tucker knowledge to people on Zoom, and we've even installed a pop-up forest in the middle of the city. Narelle's knowledge and experience is contagious, and we have seen firsthand the benefits that plants can bring. She has shown us over and again how we can befriend plants, and the meaning they can bring to our lives.

How to take this dose

If you don't already have a plant friend (i.e. a house plant), your first step is to head to your local nursery and buy one. A peace lily is a forgiving, reliable option. They always show up, day after day with their deep-green, shiny leaves and triumphant (albeit occasional) white perfect lily. A droopy peace lily comes good in a matter of hours with a little water.

Another good suggestion is a succulent. These hardy and resilient plants are great for busy or forgetful owners, requiring water just once a week. Ferns are beautiful and lush, but fragile and delicate. They need a lot of tending to, so they're better for when you're a little further along your plant friend journey.

Find a place for your plant friend where you will see it, pass it and notice it each day. Make it a little home. Perhaps it's on a windowsill for some sunlight. Maybe it's somewhere near a chair where you can sit and gaze at it.

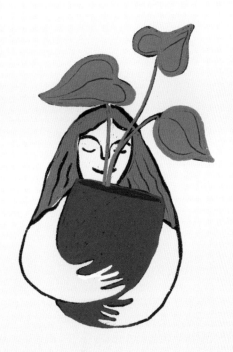

Give your plant friend a name! From here, this practice is about showing up each day to give your plant friend what it needs to survive: water, sunlight, some fresh soil occasionally, a little clipping of any brown leaves. Gently spraying the leaves with water removes dust and also feeds your plant. Noticing the changes and growth of a plant is part of this practice. Spend a moment in gratitude for the chance to keep this little plant alive, in your care.

Benefits

Research shows that spending time in nature has an immediate impact on our body, lowering our blood pressure and heart rate. It also decreases the production of cortisol, the stress hormone, and increases the production of endorphins and dopamine. One study found that adding just one small plant to a medium-sized room improves air quality by 25 per cent. Another found that plants in an indoor setting reduce feelings of anger and hostility by 44 per cent.

Taking a moment each day to tend to a plant, watering it, spraying the leaves, checking its growth and health, can help to grow our sense of kindness towards living things, including ourselves! It can remind us that every living thing needs tender loving care. It can foster a sense of purpose, as this little plant friend relies on us to stay alive. The daily tending can be a little anchor in your day.

Restore

Bowerbird

TIME NEEDED

15 minutes

MATERIALS

- Pockets
- A natural space,
  such as a bushy path,
  beach or garden

I find it almost impossible to go on a bushwalk or stroll by the sea and not come home with at least one rock, shell, mottled leaf, feather or seed pod. It's compulsive! I think in some way coming home with a small piece of the natural world in my pocket helps keep me connected to it when I'm not in it. I have piles of rocks everywhere and I rearrange them as if I'm a bowerbird all the time, occasionally sending them back to where they came from, only to replenish them again later. *Lizzie*

How to take this dose

Bowerbirds are native to Australia and are renowned for their unique courtship behaviour. The males create impressive displays of brightly coloured objects that they have collected, from shells, leaves and flowers to coins, clothing pegs and even pieces of glass. When laid together, these things no longer look like random bits of rubbish, but a bold, colourful, eye-pleasing sculpture.

Begin by spending some time (perhaps 10 minutes) tuning in to the smallest details of the ground you're standing on. It could be a forest floor, sand or grass. Without trying to reach a particular outcome, allow small things to call out to you – perhaps it's a leaf with yellow blotches, an empty seed pod or a forgotten bit of rubbish. Collect a couple of items that somehow connect to one another, either by colour, shape or purpose. Be mindful of what you collect, taking only one or two things to avoid disturbing habitats. And if you do see rubbish, pick it up and put it in the bin!

Bring your items home and arrange them in a way that pleases you, or make a small ephemeral artwork where you are. (Note that if you are in a national park, you cannot take anything home with you, so you can arrange what you've collected on site.)

Benefits

Research shows that spending time in nature has an immediate impact on our body, lowering our blood pressure and heart rate. Even the scent of plants can help reduce the production of cortisol, the stress hormone, and increase endorphins and dopamine.

The act of choosing items to make a little collection can help contain our worries and bring us into dialogue with our innate tastes – what things we like, which ones catch our eye, etc. The items don't have to carry any great meaning or story, they can simply be little items of delight.

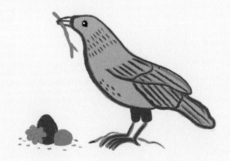

Restore

Box of Things

MEDIUM

Crafting & Making

TIME NEEDED

15 minutes

MATERIALS

● **A cardboard box**
● **Materials to decorate your box of things**

This practice is inspired by an exercise from a book by internationally acclaimed choreographer and dancer Twyla Tharp, *The Creative Habit: Learn it and use it for life* (2003).

How to take this dose

✳ Begin by decorating your box however you like – keep it simple or make it fancy. This box is a place to collect ideas for a project you've been thinking about. Over a few weeks, fill it with items that inspire you.

✳ For example, if you'd like to design a flowerbed for your garden, you might begin by looking for pictures of different flora. When you find something you like, add it to the box – maybe a dried flower or a packet of seeds, or a book on gardening.

✳ The goal is to build a collection of things. It's a little like a real-life Pinterest board.

✳ Bring out the box whenever you want to be inspired or reminded of your creative idea.

Benefits

Collecting things is a creative process. In the art world, it's called curation – carefully selecting things to group together. You write the rules when curating your box, helping discover what brings you joy or delight.

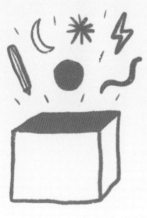

Restore

Draw Yourself as a Dwelling

MEDIUM

Mark Making

TIME NEEDED

Start with 10 minutes

MATERIALS

- **A comfy spot**
- **A piece of A4 or A5 paper**
- **Something to draw with (coloured pencils, charcoal, watercolours, markers, etc.)**
- **A timer (optional)**

This practice was shared with us by painter, artist and art therapist Sally Ann Conwell. Sally Ann facilitated one of our programs that ran over Zoom during 2020–21 to hundreds of participants across Australia.

How to take this dose

✱ Take a moment to consider this question: If you were a dwelling right now, what would you be? A log cabin? A tent? A castle, fiercely protected? A hammock under a shady tree? A leaky boat?

✱ If it's helpful, set a timer for 10 minutes.

✱ Draw your dwelling. Include any details that you find it enjoyable to spend time on.

✱ Once the timer goes off, or you're happy with your work, look at your creation.

Benefits

This practice can be a useful reminder that we can create places of safekeeping for ourselves. It can help us to remember that we are always changing and that feelings pass. Our dwelling today will likely look completely different tomorrow.

Drawing lowers our cortisol and regulates our nervous system into our Window of Tolerance (see page 121).

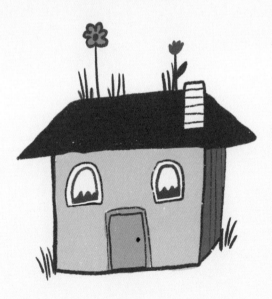

Restore

Comfort Biscuits

Makes approximately
30 biscuits

TIME NEEDED

35 minutes
(including baking)

MATERIALS

- 280 g (10 oz) butter
- 375 g (2½ cups) plain (all-purpose) flour
- 1 teaspoon baking powder
- 1 teaspoon sea salt flakes
- 115 g (½ cup firmly packed) brown sugar
- 110 g (½ cup) white sugar
- 2 teaspoons vanilla extract
- 2 eggs
- 60 g (½ cup) rolled oats
- 265 g (1½ cups) chocolate chips
- Baking trays
- Baking paper or baking mats
- A saucepan
- An oven and stovetop
- A bowl and spoon

This recipe for Comfort Biscuits comes from our friend, farmer Fiona Walmsley, who lives and works at Buena Vista Farm on the South Coast in New South Wales. Her book, *From Scratch*, features 200 handmade pantry essentials and other life-affirming kitchen miracles. She taught us how to make these delicious and comforting bickies during a retreat we ran in the forest in 2016.

How to take this dose

Brown Butter Bickies

When you can make a perfectly good biscuit with ordinary butter, is there really any point melting and browning butter and waiting for it to solidify again before turning it into bickies? Time is money and all that? Is it really worth the effort?

OH YES! Yes, it is. It is 100 per cent worth the effort.

When you brown the butter, it caramelises. It gives the bickies a wonderful crispness, butteriness and caramelness. SO GOOD! Take the time, and you'll love the result.

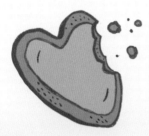

Method

* Put the butter in a small saucepan over medium heat and cook, stirring the whole time, for 2 minutes or until the butter melts and turns a caramel colour. Remove the pan from the heat and scrape the butter (including any brown bits) into a bowl. Put it in the fridge until it solidifies, effectively to room temperature – which will take about 1½ hours.
* Preheat your oven to 180°C (350°F) and line three baking trays with baking paper or baking mats.
* In a medium bowl, whisk the flour, baking powder and salt.
* In the bowl of a stand mixer fitted with the paddle attachment (you can also use hand beaters or mix it by hand), beat the chilled brown butter and both sugars at medium speed for 2 minutes or until light and fluffy. Add the vanilla and beat until smooth. Add the eggs, one at a time, beating well.
* Gently fold in the flour mixture and rolled oats with a wooden spoon, then fold in the chocolate chips.
* Roll the dough into balls approximately the size of a golf ball (or larger, if you like) between clean wet hands. Place them on the trays, allowing for spreading. Continue until all the dough has been rolled.
* Place the trays in the oven and bake for 13–15 minutes or until the biscuits are golden. If you prefer soft and chewy biscuits, take them out earlier.
* They'll store well in a sealed jar for about 4 weeks. (As if they'd last that long!)

Benefits

Baking engages all of our senses, especially taste, touch and smell. It can also spark nostalgia. When we cook or bake, we're often recreating positive experiences or happy memories. It can be a mindful and creative practice that can help bring us into the present moment through engaging with and assembling ingredients.

Cooking something simple can be a great grounding practice. Following a recipe requires us to go step by step. There is repetitive movement and action in stirring, folding, chopping and kneading. At the end of it, we have something delicious to eat and share. This can bring a sense of accomplishment, purpose, pride and inspiration for more baking adventures.

Concertina Drawing

TIME NEEDED

Start with 20 minutes

MATERIALS

- A piece of A4 paper
- A pair of scissors
- Tape
- Something to draw with (coloured pencils, charcoal, watercolours, markers, etc.)
- A timer (optional)

This practice combines two of my personal favourite things: walking in nature and quick sketch drawing. It is a rather beautiful thing to do, and I like to make my little concertina notebook, pack it along with some drawing pencils, and take myself out for a bushwalk. I then find a spot to stop and do some pretty quick, quiet sketches that become a little memento of the walk when they are in this cute little makeshift booklet. *Caitlin*

How to take this dose

✳ Fold the piece of paper lengthways down the middle, then tear or cut it along the fold to make two strips.

✳ Fold each strip into thirds, alternating the folds to the front and back.

✳ Join and tape the strips in the middle. You should end up with a folded concertina booklet with six sections to draw in.

✳ Find a place to sit somewhere that has a view.

✳ Set a timer for 10 minutes and quickly sketch one thing in each section. It could be a particular tree, then a rock, perhaps a clump of bushes. The idea here is to draw simple lines. You can use both sides of the paper, depending on what you are working with (it is trickier to do this with paint!).

- ✱ When your timer goes off, look at the rough sketches you've drawn.
- ✱ Spend some time going back over them, adding details, shading certain areas and even filling them with colour.
- ✱ At the end of this activity, you will have a little booklet of sketches from a moment in time.
- ✱ You can, if you like, use the other side to jot down any field notes – where you were, any wildlife you saw, things of note.

Benefits

Drawing lowers our cortisol and regulates our nervous system into our Window of Tolerance (see page 121). By sketching quickly, without precision or perfection, we can get into the flow of play.

Practising this kind of quick and rough sketching also helps us to accept the reality of imperfection. This is a really portable drawing activity that you can carry around in your pocket.

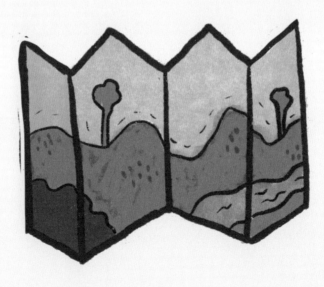

Restore

Dance in the Dark

MEDIUM

Movement
& Music

TIME NEEDED

Start with 15 minutes

MATERIALS

- Your body
- A way to play music
- Headphones
  (optional)

No Lights No Lycra is a global movement that hosts one-hour dance sessions, usually in a community hall, and for low cost. The idea is that all the lights are out, you can rock up in your tracksuit pants, and dance like no-one is watching… because no-one can see you! You can find out if there is one happening in your area. This prescription is inspired by the No Lights No Lycra movement and is your own personal version that you can do at home.

How to take this dose

This practice is simple. Find your playlist from the prescription I Dare You Not to Move (see page 170) or really any music that makes you want to dance.

Put it on. Loud. Maybe grab some headphones. It's time to dance your heart out.

Shake your arms vigorously like you are trying to dry them with the air. Feel the music in your body and try to get lost in the rhythm, releasing your energy through movement. By the end of this dance session, you want to feel puffed, out of breath and re-energised.

Benefits

Studies show that dancing can be a great nervous system regulator, particularly if we are experiencing hyperarousal (i.e. feeling highly anxious). By increasing our heart rate through cardio exercise, we can also shift into our Window of Tolerance (see page 121), which floods our system with endorphins and serotonin, and gives us a runner's high.

Dancing also releases huge amounts of energy, shifting us out of agitated states. Shaking our limbs has a similar impact, and is another practice that's recommended by somatic therapists to those experiencing the impacts of trauma, hyperactivity, anxiety and fight/flight responses.

Dancing also grounds us in our body, disrupting our busy brain. And when we combine it with music, which lights up both right and left brain, it makes this a really powerful but simple dose of creative medicine.

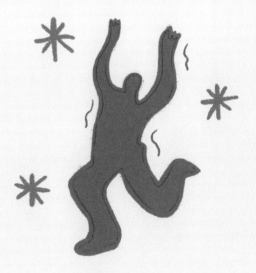

Restore

Every Seven Days

TIME NEEDED

30 minutes

MATERIALS

- A natural space,
  e.g. a beach, forest,
  park or garden (this
  also works well in an
  urban environment)

Julie Paterson is a painter, printmaker and designer of textiles. She developed this practice while, like all of us during lockdown, experiencing a sense of disconnection and anxiety. Every Seven Days is an impermanent art practice for everyone. It was set up with the aim of helping people rediscover the creative joy they used to feel, sometimes as long ago as primary school. It's designed to enhance mental health, reduce stress, boost creativity and cognitive function, and strengthen a sense of connection with nature and community.

How to take this dose

Take a quiet – silent if possible – 30-minute walk in nature, around a garden or in a park. Gather found materials (fallen or discarded things, nothing picked or nicked), such as leaves, flowers, feathers, even bottle caps or other pieces of rubbish. Contemplate a theme you would like to respond to, such as 'circle'. In this instance, you might consider the moon, the sun or the earth and create a circular artwork.

Choosing a quiet spot, use the materials you've gathered to mindfully create an ephemeral composition. There are no rules. Simply create whatever you feel inspired to.

This artwork isn't meant to last, and there can be something very grounding in that.

'Beautiful things don't last,' says Julie. 'Climate change, the pandemic, wedge politics… so many things feel tenuous and uncertain. Bleak, even. But we don't have to give in to that feeling if we take action. We can make something, we can connect with nature and each other, we can reduce stress and increase resilience, and we can be part of a supportive community.'

If you want to, take a photo of your work when you're finished. This is a lovely practice to do once a week – every seven days. You can check out @everysevendays on Instagram to see examples of this practice from people around the world.

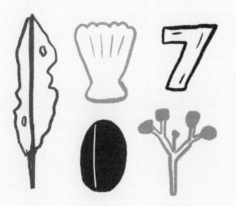

Benefits

Contemporary neuroscience has identified that creativity, nature and community all contribute to strong mental health, so now, more than ever, we believe we need this! Every Seven Days is a great tool that helps people relax into the experience of their own creativity.

Walking around our neighbourhood can help build a sense of belonging. It is also a great activity for our nervous system as well as our physical health. This practice encourages us to connect with nature, helping us to increase our curiosity and tune in to the details of what is around us during our quiet walk.

By finding materials that speak to a particular theme, we are able to flex our creative muscle in a really low-risk, low-stakes way. We are creating something, then leaving it behind, to be washed away, or picked at by birds. It can help release the grip of perfectionism and control, remembering that we can make something entirely new next time.

Restore

Make a Garden

TIME NEEDED

30–60 minutes

MATERIALS

- A 200 mm (8 inch) pot
- Potting mix
- Four different types of seedlings (you might like to select a couple of perennial herbs such as parsley, oregano, thyme or chives, and team them with a flowering companion plant, such as native daisies or violets, to bring in the helpful pollinators)
- A trowel (optional)
- Mulch (this could be leaf litter, sugar cane mulch or bark chips, or even shredded paper or cardboard)

We have had the excellent fortune of working closely with permaculture garden designer and horticulturist Narelle Happ for an entire decade. She brings a galaxy of expertise on plants, soil and design in a way that injects warmth, play and fun into the gardening process. She's guided hundreds of people in plunging their hands deep into earth, tending to flowering plants and herbs, and cheering us on as we all find ways to bring gardens into our lives, even in a tiny pot by the front door.

This prescription invites you to start your own garden – even a pot on the kitchen bench counts!

How to take this dose

* Start by grabbing your pot and potting mix, along with your seedlings.
* Using your hands or a spade, fill the pot with potting mix right to the top and water well.
* Play around with different arrangements and decide where to plant the seedlings.
* Once you like the arrangement, dig a hole and remove a seedling from its container.

* Place the seedling into the hole and fill it up with soil. Make sure to pat the soil down gently to secure the plant.
* Continue planting the seedlings to fill your pot.
* Give the plants a good soak with water. Add mulch to a depth of 5 cm (2 inches), leaving a small gap around each stem. Place the pot in a sunny position such as a back step or balcony.
* Water daily or as required. You can use your finger to test if the soil is moist. If it is, water your pot the following day.

Benefits

Gardening has been shown to actively reduce feelings of stress, anxiety and depression. It can help to bring us into our Window of Tolerance (see page 121) by engaging our senses of touch, sight and smell, and later, taste!

Our connection to plants is so strong that being in the presence of a plant for just a few minutes can help decrease stress levels.

The daily tending to your potted garden is an act of care that provides a moment of connection. Watering and then harvesting edible plants also enhances our connection with the world around us.

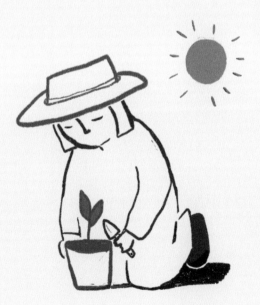

Restore

Mixtape

TIME NEEDED

Start with 30 minutes

MATERIALS

- Your eyes and ears
- A music app such as Spotify, Apple Music, BandCamp
- A device to create your playlist on

Making playlists is one of my favourite things, and also one I love making for other people. In the olden days, the 1980s and 1990s, it was actually on cassette, where you would have to do the analogue physical act of pressing record and pause for each song, making that clunky bump between each transition. I still have some of those tapes, but nothing to listen to them with. One of my most treasured is a mixtape of songs made by my now husband, for when I went on a trip without him for three weeks. It was an act of such thoughtfulness, creativity and love.

Making a playlist for you or someone else can also capture a moment in time. It can be like a little hug for yourself, your own little soft blanket of songs for times when you really need the wave of beautiful music to move you, soothe you or make you feel all the feelings. *Caitlin*

How to take this dose

Think of this as a soundtrack designed to help improve your mood at any time. Perhaps your soundtrack features soft, gentle, meditative sounds, or maybe it's filled with thumping, rhythmic drum and bass tracks. It's your choice – there's no right or wrong.

Aim to create a playlist that contains 15 songs – around the length of an album. Start with one or two songs that simply put you in a different headspace when you listen to them. Maybe they are uplifting. Maybe they make you smile. Maybe they are attached to a good memory or moment that you'll never forget.

Play around with listening to different songs and then adding the ones that resonate to your playlist. If you are a little lost, most music platforms will recommend songs, e.g. 'If you like this song, then you might like that one', etc. Give your playlist a name. You now have a companion for whenever you're washing the dishes, going for a walk or just lying in bed.

With the right beat, the right chord progression, the right melody, music can also pick us up off the floor. Find the music that speaks to you.

This practice also helps strengthen your taste muscle, helping you to learn what you do and don't like. You can change your mind. You can think you love a song, have it on your playlist, then mid walk-with-headphones change your mind, and guess what? You can remove it! It can be a good practice in building the idea that you can change your mind, and change it back again.

Benefits

Music is the one human experience that fires up our brains in ways that nothing else does. When we watch a movie, it's the soundtrack that gives us cues to the emotional experience of characters. Music has an incredible ability to impact how we feel. Sometimes sad, mournful or melancholic music can help us practise these emotions and feelings, allowing us a moment of release if talking just isn't cutting the mustard.

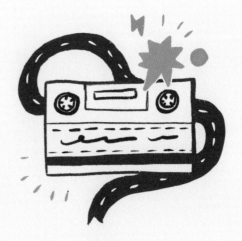

Restore

Nature Field Notes

MEDIUM

Nature &
Adventure

TIME NEEDED

Start with 20 minutes

MATERIALS

- A spot in nature
- A notebook
- A pen or pencil

I have been collecting information about what I see around me for decades. I have a stack of unfinished notebooks in a pile, with observations about places I have lived. They include snippets and sketches about the creatures I've seen, what the sun was doing, what flowers were growing or if I stumbled across something delightful. It doesn't have to be a serious scientific account, it's more about snatching a piece of information about what you see. *Lizzie*

How to take this dose

Find a comfortable place to sit outside, in nature. Spend some time just sitting quietly and observing what is happening around you. Tune in to the big things and the small; notice sounds as well as sights.

A field note simply captures little bits of information about what is around you. You might want to start by doing a quick drawing of things you see. Bird watchers use the acronym GISS – general impression of size and shape. This prescription invites you to draw anything you like, not just birds, but it can be a helpful reminder that we are recording general impressions, and not trying to create a photographic image.

Take out your notebook and pen, and write a short record of your observations, capturing this moment in time.

Benefits

Research shows that spending time in nature has an immediate impact on our body, lowering our blood pressure and our heart rate. Even the scent of plants can help reduce the production of cortisol, the stress hormone, and increase endorphins and dopamine.

Observing life like a scientist on a field trip – taking in all the small details without judging them – can also help us reflect on our own life. Just like us, birds are navigating hardship and challenges, loss and opportunity, life and death, every single day. This practice can help remind us that we, too, are creatures of the earth. We all have to make our ways finding food, building a home and creating safety in our own life experience.

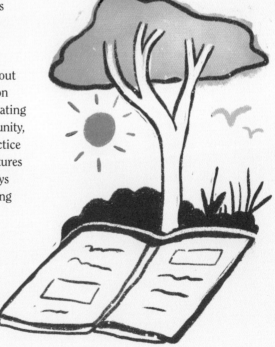

Restore

Paint to Music

TIME NEEDED

10–15 minutes

MATERIALS

- Access to a stereo or some way to listen to music
- A piece of A3 paper (or bigger)
- A paintbrush
- Paints
- A glass of water

This beautiful practice was shared with us by Australian artist Clare Thackway. During one of our first workshops around creativity as a form of therapy, we gathered 15 people in a hall by the sea. Clare arrived with a giant stack of various types of paper, paintbrushes and pots of paint. She put on a playlist and encouraged us not to talk, but to listen to the music and respond to the rhythm by making lines across a page with paint. When a track ended and a new song came on, we got a new piece of paper and a new colour of paint, and we were guided to listen and respond by making dots across the page. We did this several times until we were flowing freely in response to the music – making whatever lines, marks, spots, shapes we felt like, not overthinking the process, but working with paint and music from a gut response. It was like a meditation.

How to take this dose

Take three big breaths, in and out. Notice the tension you might feel in different parts of your body. Put on some music. Ideally, it's music that gives you energy and inspires feelings of joy, hope or excitement.

Grab your paintbrush and put a little paint on it – not much – then dip it in the water.

Start moving the brush across your paper, in time to the music. Make changes in the style of your painting according to the rhythm and melody of whatever song you're listening to.

You are not trying to make an image here. Simply tune in to the feeling of the brush moving across the page. Look at the colour spreading, the way the watery paint moves on the paper, too. Feel free to pick different colours as you go along.

Do this for as long as you are in the flow of it. At the end, you might have paper full of colour, interesting shapes and lines, and maybe even a few surprises.

Benefits

Painting to music and making repeat patterns engages the prefrontal cortex of the brain. And it helps bring us into the present moment. Listening to music can also help to regulate our nervous system. When we practise loose, free playing with paint, we can let go of perfection – it's just lines and swirls.

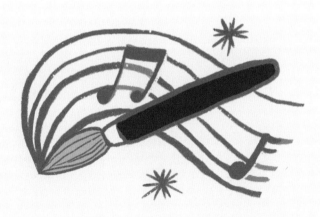

Restore

Pass It On

TIME NEEDED

5 minutes – or longer if
you're making a meal!

MATERIALS

● This will depend
on what you want to
pass on to someone.
It might be a coffee,
a meal, a playlist or
an experience, such
as a ticket to a show.
It could also be an
image of something
you find inspiring, a
poem or even a song.

Back in the early days of MakeShift, when
we didn't know how to lodge a Business
Activity Statement and we paid ourselves
in marker pens, we attended a conference
run by musician Clare Bowditch, called
Big Hearted Business. In the middle of
the conference courtyard stood a very large
tree. Over the next few days, participants
tied handwritten offerings of knowledge,
support and care to the branches like
paper leaves. The idea was that by tying
them to this 'giving tree', these 'offerings'
would continue to grow. This concept of
the giving tree has deep roots in our work.
The facilitators at MakeShift so generously
offer up their knowledge and passion as
gifts through creative activities that anyone
can do. Passing something on to someone
else works both ways, filling up both the
recipient and the giver.

How to take this dose

With intention, think about someone who
could do with a spontaneous 'gift', an act
of kindness. If you decide to make someone
a cup of tea or share a poem with them, do
it straight away. If you want to cook a meal
for someone who might need a break, then
plan ahead.

You can strengthen this dose by applying it to a stranger. Pay for the coffee of the person in the line behind you at your local cafe. Take a neighbour's bins in off the street. Help carry someone's heavy shopping bags to their car. There are a million different ways you can 'pass it on'.

Benefits

When we offer someone else an act of kindness, it releases feel-good chemicals such as serotonin, dopamine and oxytocin in our brain. It can also distract us from our own worries and help foster our curiosity by getting us thinking about another person and what might bring a smile to their face. In fact, volunteering has been shown through research to improve people's senses of self, purpose and identity, and there are even some community groups that prescribe volunteering just like medicine! Finally, giving a gift to someone can enhance our sense of purpose – it's a powerful reminder that we are 'all in this together'.

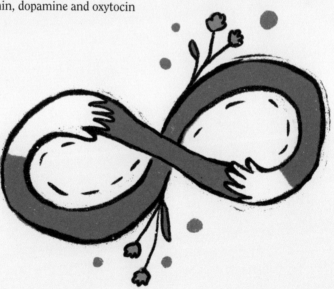

Restore

Photo Treasure Hunt

TIME NEEDED

10–30 minutes

MATERIALS

- A smartphone or camera

This activity was invented during a moment when I was up against a huge work deadline and had kids in lockdown, learning from home. What a juggle that was! In an attempt to stay with the huge document I was working on, I gave the kids my phone and a list of ten things to find around the house and outside in the garden, and told them to each take a photo of what they found. They loved it and came back for another list, and another. I managed to submit what I was working on and later MakeShift developed this into part of a workshop for adults. *Lizzie*

How to take this dose

Take yourself on a little walk. It could be around your house, street, neighbourhood or even your workplace.

Your mission is to find the list of treasures below and take a photograph of each item.

✳ Something bright pink
✳ A tiny machine
✳ A face with eyes open
✳ A piece of fruit
✳ Something with scales
✳ Something soft

* Something that could melt in the sun
* A thing you wear on your head
* A creature
* A piece of trash that might be someone else's treasure

Once you've done this, you can make up your own treasure list to challenge yourself, or others.

Benefits

Like some of the other prescriptions inviting us to take a little adventure, even if it's not far from home, this Photo Treasure Hunt can help strengthen our curiosity by taking an everyday act and making it special. This practice can open our eyes to see the familiar in new and interesting ways. By challenging ourselves to find a variety of items on our treasure hunt, we can wake up our minds, activating us to be motivated.

Photography, which is now so readily and constantly available via our smartphones, is an opportunity to be creative and find ways to use these addictive gadgets to make us feel good!

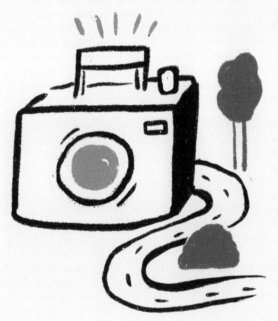

Restore

Sit Spot

TIME NEEDED

Start with 30 minutes

MATERIALS

- A cushion
- A timer

This practice was shared with us by Andrew Turbill (aka The Bird Guy) and taught to us as part of a bird language workshop retreat. In his words, the sit spot practice is 'likely as old as the human species, but I teach it as a core routine in deepening nature connection, and in seeing nature when it is in a state of not being freaked out by your human presence!'

We spent three days in the bush, experimenting with sitting quietly for long periods of time, including once in the darkness of night. We have amended Andrew's version here, but you can learn more about his work via the resources section (see page 258).

How to take this dose

The Sit Spot is a practice of observing the natural world. The intention is to return to a spot over and over, building your experiences of this place through repeat visits.

Find a spot in a natural space – this could be a garden, a forest, a wood, a pond – whatever you have access to.

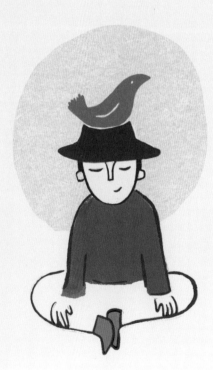

Sit on the cushion for a timed period, as still as you can. There is no need to be frozen and uncomfortable, but avoid moving around a lot.

The intention is to let nature relax – once the alarm of your presence has died down, creatures and insects relax, too. This is a beautiful opportunity to observe birds, reptiles and insects.

We might spend ten minutes in frantic conversation with ourselves: 'But I'm not seeing any birds!' 'How long has it been?' Let this part pass. We might start to notice things that we didn't see at first. We might notice sounds that weren't obvious at first. We might get a front-row seat to some birds in conversation.

Stay curious. This isn't about knowing what bird you hear, what tree you see. It's about tuning in to the busy, teeming life in nature that often passes us by, and seeing what is really there, not just what we think is there.

You can start with setting a timer so that you know when 30 minutes is up. You might like to sit for longer.

Benefits

Spending time in nature helps lower our blood pressure and heart rate. It can also increase the production of endorphins and dopamine, while decreasing cortisol, the stress hormone.

When we are still and watchful, we mirror the practice of mindfulness meditation, but by observing creatures, plants and behaviours we take the focus off ourselves and transfer it onto something else. Observing the world in this way can help us reflect on our own. This can also restore our capacity for 'soft fascination' – to notice detail without focused concentration. Birds are navigating life and death, hardship and challenge, loss and opportunity every single day. This practice can help remind us that we, too, are animals, creatures of the earth. And one day you may just make a new friend through gaining the trust of a wild creature that routinely starts coming closer and closer to you, or even landing or crawling on you. Wild trust can be life-changing!

Restore

Slow Stitch

TIME NEEDED

10–30 minutes

MATERIALS

- A piece of fabric
  (e.g. calico or cotton)
- Some thread in
  different colours
- A sewing needle

This stitching practice was shared with us
by MakeShift facilitator Michele Elliot, who
you met on page 144. Michele has taught
hundreds of people the meditative practice
of slow stitching, or *kantha*. Originating
on the east coast of India, *kantha* is a great
creative practice that can help us slow down
and return to a state of calm.

How to take this dose

Begin by threading your needle
✳ Cut a piece of thread about 35–40 cm
  (14–16 inches) long.
✳ Squeeze the thread strands together
  at one end between your thumb and
  pointer finger.
✳ Feed the thread through the eye of
  the needle.
✳ Tie a double knot at the end of the thread.

Start your stitch
✳ Starting about 1 cm (½ inch) in from the
  edge of the fabric, push the needle from
  the back to the front of the fabric, then
  from the front to the back, and pull the
  thread through.
✳ Keep stitching in a straight line, taking
  the thread in and out of the fabric to create
  a row of stitches.

* Try to keep the cloth flat, and avoid pulling the stitches too tight. Remember that the stitches don't all have to be the same size.
* When you finish the piece of thread, bring the needle through to the back of the fabric and tie a double knot.
* Continue on from where you left off with a new piece of thread.

Create a pattern

* Take a different coloured thread from your kit and start stitching next to your original pattern, but this time stitch in the opposite direction. Make a few rows – they can be different lengths.
* Take another different coloured thread and stitch across the original lines in the opposite direction. You should end up with a piece of fabric adorned with colourful cross-hatched lines.

Benefits

Stitching, like many craft activities, is a meditative practice, as we are required to do an action over and over. This can bring us into the zone of play and flow, allowing us to lose track of time and quieten down our brain.

By literally being able to watch as the stitches, one by one, add up to making lines, patterns and shapes, we are reminded that we can shift from one place to another, little by little, one small step at a time. Small actions can add up to big outcomes.

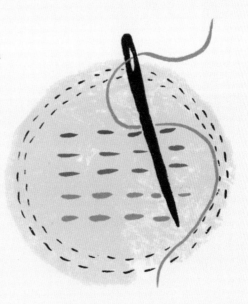

Restore

A Slow-motion Walk

MEDIUM

Movement

TIME NEEDED

20 minutes

MATERIALS

- A timer

Our friend and collaborator Emma Saunders is a choreographer and dancer who has worked with diverse groups of people in community, performance and education settings. One sunny Sunday morning, we joined Emma on a soccer field on Dharawal Country for something she calls Slow-motion Walking. It took us half an hour to walk from one side of the field to the other. During that time, our moods ranged from bored and daydreamy, to focused and impatient, and eventually reflective and calm. The activity left us feeling like we'd just had a giant sleep.

Slow-motion Walking has been used as a training tool within performative practices since the 1960s, and was introduced to Emma by New York–based choreographer Miguel Gutierrez.

How to take this dose

This exercise is a meditation in slowing down, planting your feet on the earth and walking in slow motion.

Find an outdoor space that has an area of about 10 metres (around 30 feet). It should ideally be flat and free to walk on.

Set a timer and begin walking. The idea is to walk so slowly that it takes 20 minutes to walk around 10 metres. Notice thoughts come and go in your head, and the feelings that come up.

You don't need to practise mindfulness or clear your thoughts, or stick with a breathing rhythm. The only rule is to keep the slow-motion pace.

Benefits

Forcing ourselves to literally slow down can help give us perspective on how much we rush through our lives. Bringing this slowness to the simple practice of walking helps to bring awareness to the strength and grace of our legs. While our body might naturally want to hurry up, we must accept the challenge of slowing down.

With our smartphones readily available to provide constant distraction, we never have the opportunity to experience boredom. This practice can help us cycle through the many thoughts we encounter when we are forced to wait.

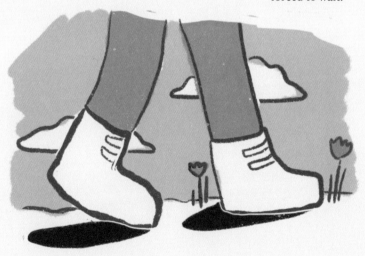

Combined

Treatment Plans

A series of three-week creative prescription plans
to build habits, confidence and practice.

MEDIUM

Various

Dose of Drawing

This treatment plan is intended to help
build a habit of drawing. These practices
are all portable and can become a reliable
tool to support you, whether you need some
immediate relief or are working to keep
up a short and easy drawing practice, all
the way to having a beautiful process to
explore when time permits.

1. Apply first aid with a Relief Remedy
Blind Contour Drawing (page 168)
Time: 1–3 minutes each day

2. Time for a Recharge
Hirameki (page 198)
A great plan is to make five to seven sheets of
hirameki 'blobs' with watercolour or acrylic
paint, or chalk pastels mixed with water, so
you have some ready to go.
*Time: A couple of times a week in Weeks 2 and 3,
alongside your Blind Contour Drawing practice*

3. Now for some Restoration
Concertina Drawing (page 228)
*Time: Daily in Week 3, alongside
your Blind Contour Drawing practice*

A Case of Curiosity

This treatment plan is intended to help
foster and build the muscle of curiosity.

1. Apply first aid with a Relief Remedy
Write What You See (page 176)
Time: 10 minutes a day, as required

2. Time for a Recharge
Your Perfect Day (page 204)
Time: 20–30 minutes, once a week

3. Now for some Restoration
Photo Treasure Hunt (page 244)
Time: 10–30 minutes, once a week

A Nature Plan

This treatment plan intends to help foster
a practice of nature connection.

1. Apply first aid with a Relief Remedy
Owl Eyes (page 172)
Time: 2 minutes, as required

2. Time for a Recharge
Tiny and Giant, All at Once (page 216)
Time: 20 minutes, once a week

3. Now for some Restoration
Sit Spot (page 246)
Time: 30–60 minutes, once a week

Making a Move

This treatment plan intends to help foster
a practice of creative movement.

1. Apply first aid with a Relief Remedy
I Dare You Not to Move (page 170)
Time: 20 minutes, as required

2. Time for a Recharge
Brain Dance (page 218)
Time: 10 minutes, daily

3. Now for some Restoration
Dance in the Dark (page 230)
Time: 15 minutes, once a week

Treatment Plans

A series of three-week creative prescription plans
to build habits, confidence and practice.

Combined

MEDIUM

Various

A Dose of Self-Compassion

This treatment plan is intended to help foster
and build the muscle of curiosity.

1. Apply first aid with a Relief Remedy
Compassion Palming (page 162)
Time: 5 minutes a day, as required

2. Time for a Recharge
Glimmer Hunting (page 212)
Time: 5–10 minutes, as required

3. Now for some Restoration
Draw Yourself as a Dwelling (page 225)
Time: 30 minutes

Strengthening Safekeeping

This treatment plan is intended to
strengthen and build capacity for
safekeeping.

1. Apply first aid with a Relief Remedy
Six Directions (page 184)
Time: 2 minutes a day, as required

Five Senses Reboot (page 160)
Time: 1 minute, as required

2. Time for a Recharge
Bilateral Drawing (page 188)
Time: 5–10 minutes, as required

Visual Poetry (page 208)
Time: 15–30 minutes

3. Now for some Restoration
Box of Things (page 224)
Time: 30 minutes

A Playfulness Prescription

This treatment plan is intended to strengthen and build playfulness.

1. Apply first aid with a Relief Remedy
Four Faces (page 166)
Time: 2 minutes a day

2. Time for a Recharge
Hirameki (page 198)
Time: 10–15 minutes, once a week

Cut and Paste (page 214)
Time: 15–30 minutes

3. Now for some Restoration
Every Seven Days (page 232)
Time: 30 minutes, once a week

Inch by Inch

This treatment plan is also intended to strengthen and build playfulness.

1. Apply first aid with a Relief Remedy
Mindful Mindless Mark Making (page 164)
Time: 2 minutes a day, as required

2. Time for a Recharge
Making Pompoms (page 206)
Time: 10–15 minutes

3. Now for some Restoration
Nature Field Notes (page 238)
Time: 30 minutes, once a week

Slow Stitch (page 248)
Time: 20 minutes, as required

Hidden Track

In the field of recorded music, a hidden track (sometimes called a ghost track, secret track or unlisted track) is a song or a piece of audio that has been placed on a CD, audio cassette, LP record or other recorded medium in such a way as to avoid detection by the casual listener.

Friends. Thanks for taking this journey with us.

We hope it continues, and that creative practice takes up a little more space in your life. Because, remember, it's good for us!

Let us say thank you to artists and creatives. They bring us glimmers and mountains of joy through songs, plays, books, sculptures, poems and dances. Their role is a vital heartbeat for all our lives. In a way this book is our love song to you, dear artists.

And finally, before we go, we thought we'd leave this little list of really great things that we should all be doing as much as we can. They are tiny little droplets of glimmery goodness, micro resets of our nervous system, and add up to giving ourselves some tiny moments of self-care, rest and radical restoration, every single day.

They don't need much explanation. Go forth and pat furry things with your shoes off.

* Go outside.
* Pat a creature!
* Splash your face with cold water when you wake up.
* Don't be a d!*k to your future self.
* Sit around a fire when you can.
* Read a book.
* Take your freaking shoes off.
* Brush your teeth outside.
* Look at the moon.
* Look at art.
* Listen to music you've never heard before.
* Send a postcard.
* Drink water.

Resources

Below is a list of resources that we have found to be illuminating and valuable on the topics of creative first aid, trauma, neuroscience, psychology, connection, First Nations wisdom, and nature medicine.

Books

Anchored: How to befriend your nervous system using polyvagal theory by Deb Dana

The Artist's Way by Julia Cameron

The Body Keeps the Score: Brain, mind, and body in the healing of trauma by Bessel van der Kolk

The Creative Act: A way of being by Rick Rubin

The Dreaming Path: Indigenous thinking to change your life by Paul Callaghan with Uncle Paul Gordon

Habit Stacking: 97 small life changes that take five minutes or less by S.J. Scott

The Hidden Life of Trees: What they feel, how they communicate – discoveries from a secret world by Peter Wohlleben

Hoodie Economics: Changing our systems to value what matters by Jack Manning Bancroft

Lost Connections: Why you're depressed and how to find hope by Johann Hari

The Luminous Solution by Charlotte Wood

The Myth of Normal: Trauma, illness and healing in a toxic culture by Gabor Maté with Daniel Maté

Nature, Our Medicine: How the natural world sustains us by Dimity Williams

Play: How it shapes the brain, opens the imagination, and invigorates the soul by Stuart Brown, MD with Christopher Vaughan

The Pocket Guide to the Polyvagal Theory: The transformative power of feeling safe by Stephen W. Porges

Polyvagal Exercises for Safety and Connection by Deb Dana

The Polyvagal Theory: Neurophysiological foundations of emotions, attachment, communication, self-regulation by Stephen W. Porges

The Post-Traumatic Growth Guidebook: Practical mind–body tools to heal trauma, foster resilience and awaken your potential by Arielle Schwartz

Sand Talk: How indigenous thinking can save the world by Tyson Yunkaporta

Underland by Robert Macfarlane

24-hour Crisis Support

Australia
Lifeline: 13 11 14
Beyond Blue: 1300 22 4636

New Zealand
Lifeline: 0800 543 354
Healthline: 0800 611 116

MakeShift Artists

Marcelo Baez
marcelobaez.com

Sarah Ball
sarahball.com.au

Angie Cass
angiecass.com

Sally Ann Conwell
@sallyannconwell

Michele Elliot
micheleelliot.com

Helena Fox
helenafoxauthor.com
How it Feels to Float (2019) and
The Quiet and The Loud (2023)
are published by Pan Macmillan

Narelle Happ
agardenforlife.com.au

Linda Kennedy
future-black.com

Kiara Mucci
@themuccibird

Nooky
wearewarriors.com.au

Julie Paterson
juliepaterson.com.au

Therese Petre
peacharoo.co

Emma Saunders
@emmasaundersemma

Kirli Saunders (OAM)
kirlisaunders.com

Elana Stone
elanastone.com.au

Clare Thackway
clarethackway.com

Andrew Turbill
andrewthebirdguy.com

Fiona Walmsley
buenavistafarm.com.au/author/
fiona-walmsley

Melinda Young
melindayoung.net

Notes

Introduction: Our story

1. The term 'grumpy struggle' was initially coined by Janet Burroway and explained further by Charlotte Wood. Burroway, J., *A Story Larger than my Own: Women writers look back on their lives and careers*, Chicago: University of Chicago Press, 2014; Wood, C., *The Luminous Solution*, Sydney: Allen & Unwin, 2021
2. Full Stop Australia has been supporting people impacted by sexual, domestic and family violence since 1971. They are an accredited, nationally focused, not-for-profit organisation providing support, education, advocacy and training to the community. Full Stop Australia, 2023 <fullstop.org.au>
3. 'Vicarious trauma' describes 'the cumulative effects of exposure to information about traumatic events and experiences, potentially leading to distress, dissatisfaction, hopelessness and serious mental and physical health problems'. Monash Gender and Family Violence Prevention Centre, 'Best Practice Guidelines: Supporting the wellbeing of family violence workers during times of emergency and crisis', 17 May 2021 <doi.org/10.26180/14605005.v1>
4. From the late 1960s to the early 1980s, Brisbane experienced what's known as the Brisbane Social Protests – a swell of activism in response to the Vietnam War, the lack of recognition of Indigenous land sovereignty and rights, and of the right to protest under the ultra-conservative and famously corrupt state government led by Joh Bjelke-Petersen.
5. Khan & Giurca et al., 2023, 'Social prescribing around the world', National Academy for Social Prescribing, p. 47 <socialprescribingacademy. org.uk/media/1yeoktid/social-prescribing-around-the-world. pdf>
6. Hotz, J., 'How Strangers Use Storytelling to Help Others – and Themselves', *Time*, 4 February 2022 <time.com/6144918/ storytelling-circles-benefits-pandemic-anxiety>
7. Jordan, A., Searle, S. & Dunphy, K., 'The dance of life with Aboriginal and Torres Strait Islander peoples', *Dance Therapy Collections*, 2017, no. 4, pp. 51–66
8. Porges, S.W., *The Pocket Guide to the Polyvagal Theory: The transformative power of feeling safe*, New York, NY: Norton Professional Books, 2017
9. Brown, S. with Vaughan, C., *Play: How it shapes the brain, opens the imagination, and invigorates the soul*, New York, NY: Avery, 2009

Chapter 1: Creative First Aid

1. Murray, W.H., *Mountaineering in Scotland*, Riverside, CA: Dent, 1947
2. Silva, F. & Azimitabar, M., 'It brought me a smile they couldn't take from me', *Law Society Journal*, 1 July 2022, vol. 1 no. 1, pp. 124–7
3. Bancroft, J.M., *Hoodie Economics: Changing our systems to value what matters*, Melbourne: Hardie Grant, 2023
4. Such as the Sharing Culture Project. Sharing Culture Project, accessed 1 August 2023 <sharingculture.info>
5. Brown, S. with Vaughan, C., *Play: How it shapes the brain, opens the imagination, and invigorates the soul*, New York, NY: Avery, 2009
6. Brown, S., *Play*, p. 42
7. Brown, S., 2023, The Institute for Play <nifplay.org>
8. Proyer, R.T., 'The well-being of playful adults: Adult playfulness, subjective well-being, physical well-being, and the pursuit of enjoyable activities', *European Journal of Humour Research*, January 2013, vol. 1 no. 1, pp. 84–98
9. Csikszentmihalyi, M., *Flow: The psychology of optimal experience*, New York, NY: Harper & Row, 1990
10. Le, N. & Savige, J., 1 October 2020, 'Chops and surrender': Nam Le Interviews Jaya Savige, Cordite Poetry Review <cordite.org.au/ interviews/le-savige/5>
11. Johnson, S., 20 December 2022, *Adjacent Possible: Little Beginnings Everywhere*, Substack <adjacentpossible.substack. com/p/little-beginnings-everywhere>
12. Gilbert, P. & Woodyatt, L., 'An Evolutionary Approach to Shame-Based Self-Criticism, Self-Forgiveness, and Compassion', in Woodyatt, L. et al. (eds), *Handbook of the Psychology of Self-Forgiveness*, Cham: Springer, 2017, pp. 29–41 <doi.org/10.1007/978-3-319-60573-9_3>
13. Macfarlane, R., *Underland*, New York, NY: W.W. Norton, 2019, p. 79
14. van der Kolk, B.A., *The Body Keeps the Score: Brain, mind, and body in the healing of trauma*, New York, NY: Viking, 2014
15. van der Kolk, B.A., *The Body Keeps the Score*

16. Tedeschi, R.G. & Calhoun, L.G., 'Posttraumatic Growth: Conceptual Foundations and Empirical Evidence', *Psychological Inquiry*, 2004, vol. 15 no. 1, pp. 1–18 <doi.org/10.1207/s15327965pli1501_01>

Chapter 2: Creativity as Medicine

1. Davies, C., Knuiman, M. & Rosenberg, M., 'The art of being mentally healthy: a study to quantify the relationship between recreational arts engagement and mental well-being in the general population', *BMC Public Health*, 5 January 2016, vol. 16 no. 1, pp. 1–10 <doi.org/10.1186/s12889-015-2672-7>

2. Whitaker, R., *Anatomy of an Epidemic: Magic bullets, psychiatric drugs, and the astonishing rise of mental illness in America*, New York, NY: Crown Publishers, 2010

3. Gopnik, A., *The Philosophical Baby: What children's minds tell us about truth, love, and the meaning of life*, New York, NY: Random House, 1998

4. MakeShift, November 2021, *ReMind Creativity on Prescription: Project evaluation report*, p. 29 <makeshift.org.au/post/hopefor-the-future-how-our-creativefirst-aid-program-transformedpeoples-lives>

5. Burns, P. & Van Der Meer, R., 'Happy Hookers: findings from an international study exploring the effects of crochet on wellbeing', *Perspectives in Public Health*, May 2021, vol. 141 no. 3, pp. 149–57 <doi.org/10.1177/1757913920911961>

6. Gerdes, M.E. et al., 'Reducing Anxiety with Nature and Gardening (RANG): Evaluating the Impacts of Gardening and Outdoor Activities on Anxiety among U.S. Adults during the COVID-19 Pandemic', *International Journal of Environmental Research and Public Health*, 22 April 2022, vol. 19 no. 9 <doi.org/10.3390/ijerph19095121>

7. Wohlleben, P., *The Hidden Life of Trees: What they feel, how they communicate – discoveries from a secret world*, Melbourne: Black Inc., 2016

8. Hammoud, R. et al., 'Smartphone-based ecological momentary assessment reveals mental health benefits of birdlife', *Scientific Reports*, 27 October 2022, vol. 12 no. 17589 <doi.org/10.1038/s41598-022-20207-6>

9. Braun Janzen, T. et al., 'A Pilot Study Investigating the Effect of Music-Based Intervention on Depression and Anhedonia', *Frontiers in Psychology*, 8 May 2019, vol. 10 no. 1038 <doi.org/10.3389/fpsyg.2019.01038>

10. Gustavson, D.E. et al., 'Mental health and music engagement: review, framework, and guidelines for future studies', *Translational Psychiatry*, 22 June 2021, vol. 11 no. 370 <doi.org/10.1038/s41398-021-01483-8>

11. MacKinnon, L. with Perry, B., 'The Neurosequential Model of Therapeutics: An Interview with Bruce Perry', *Australian and New Zealand Journal of Family Therapy*, vol. 33 no. 3, September 2012, pp. 210–18 <doi.org/10.1017/aft.2012.26>

12. Steinberg, S., 'Let's Dance: A Holistic Approach to Treating Veterans With Posttraumatic Stress Disorder', *Federal Practitioner*, July 2016, vol. 33 no. 7, pp. 44–9 <pubmed.ncbi.nlm.nih.gov/30766191>

13. Robens, S. et al., 'Effects of Choir Singing on Mental Health: Results of an Online Cross-sectional Study', *Journal of Voice*, 3 July 2022 <doi.org/10.1016/j.jvoice.2022.06.003>

14. Petrie, K.J. et al., 'Effect of Written Emotional Expression on Immune Function in Patients With Human Immunodeficiency Virus Infection: A Randomized Trial', *Psychosomatic Medicine*, March 2004, vol. 66 no. 2, pp. 272–5 <doi.org/10.1097/01.psy.0000116782.49850.d3>

15. Kaimal, G., Ray, K. & Muniz, J., 'Reduction of Cortisol Levels and Participants' Responses Following Art Making', *Art Therapy*, 23 May 2016, vol. 33 no. 2, pp. 74–80 <doi.org/10.1080/07421656.2016.1166832>

16. Gullotta, D. & Boydell, K., Black Dog Institute with Art Gallery of NSW, 2023, *Culture Dose* <blackdoginstitute.org.au/research-centres/culture-dose>

17. Zoom interview: Katherine Boydell and Caitlin Marshall, November 2022

18. Estevao, C. et al., 'Scaling-up Health-Arts Programmes: the largest study in the world bringing arts-based mental health interventions into a national health service', *BJPsych Bulletin*, February 2021, vol. 45 no. 1, pp. 32–9 <doi.org/10.1192/bjb.2020.122>

19. Starlight Children's Foundation, 2020, *Captain Starlight* <starlight.org.au/about-us/what-we-do/captain-starlight>

20. Starlight Children's Foundation, 2020, *Family and Hospital Partners Impact Study*

21. Davies, C.R. et al., 'The art of being healthy: A qualitative study to develop a thematic framework for understanding

the relationship between health and the arts', *BMJ Open*, 25 April 2014, vol. 4 no. 4 <doi.org/10.1136/bmjopen-2014-004790>

22. Davies, C.R. et al., 'The art of being healthy'

23. Flett, J.A.M. et al., 'Sharpen Your Pencils: Preliminary Evidence that Adult Coloring Reduces Depressive Symptoms and Anxiety', *Creativity Research Journal*, 2 October 2017, vol. 29 no. 4, pp. 409–16 <doi.org/10.1080/10400419.2017.1376505>

24. Mental Health First Aid Australia, 2023 <mhfa.com.au>

25. Australian Institute of Health and Welfare (AIHW), *Mental Health Services in Australia: Stress and trauma*, Canberra: AIHW, 2022 <aihw.gov.au/reports/mental-health-services/stress-and-trauma>

26. Standard MHFA Teaching Notes, Session 1 Ed. 4, November 2022, Mental Health First Aid International

27. Australian Institute of Health and Welfare (AIHW), *Australia's Health 2014*, Canberra: AIHW, 2014 <aihw.gov.au/reports/australias-health/australias-health-2014/overview>

28. Gallup, 2 May 2023, *State of the Global Workplace: 2022 Report* <cca-global.com/content/latest/article/2023/05/state-of-the-global-workplace-2022-report-346>

29. Bower, M. et al., 'A hidden pandemic? An umbrella review of global evidence on mental health in the time of COVID-19', *Frontiers in Psychiatry*, 8 March 2023, vol. 14 <doi.org/10.3389/fpsyt.2023.1107560>

30. Australian Bureau of Statistics, 22 July 2022, *National Study of Mental Health and Wellbeing: 2020–21* <abs.gov.au/statistics/health/mental-health/national-study-mental-health-and-wellbeing/2020-21>

31. Australian Institute of Health and Welfare, 7 July 2022, *Indigenous Health and Wellbeing* <aihw.gov.au/reports/australias-health/indigenous-health-and-wellbeing>

32. The Healing Foundation, 2023 <healingfoundation.org.au>

33. LGBTIQ+ Health Australia, 13 May 2021, *Snapshot of Mental Health and Suicide Prevention Statistics for LGBTIQ+ People* <lgbtiqhealth.org.au/statistics>

34. World Health Organization (WHO), 9 March 2021, *Violence against women* <who.int/news-room/fact-sheets/detail/violence-against-women>

35. Woo, B. et al., 'The role of racial/ethnic identity in the association between racial discrimination and psychiatric disorders: A buffer or exacerbator?', *SSM Population Health*, April 2019, vol. 7 <doi.org/10.1016/j.ssmph.2019.100378>

36. Ford, J.D. et al., 'Social, cultural, and other diversity issues in the traumatic stress field', in *Posttraumatic Stress Disorder* (second edition), San Diego, CA: Academic Press, 2015, pp. 503–46

37. Australian Healthcare Index, November 2022, *Report 4: Australian Healthcare Index November 2022* <australianhealthcareindex.com.au/australian-healthcare-index-november-2022>

38. Wallis, K.A., Donald, M. & Moncrieff, J., 'Antidepressant prescribing in general practice: "A call to action"', *Australian Journal of General Practice*, 1 December 2021, vol. 50 no. 12, pp. 954–6

39. Hari, J., *Lost Connections: Why you're depressed and how to find hope*, New York, NY: Bloomsbury, 2019

40. Schmitz, A., 'Benzodiazepines: the time for systematic change is now', *Addiction*, February 2021, vol. 116 no. 2, pp. 219–21 <doi.org/10.1111/add.15095>

41. Moncrieff, J. et al., 'The serotonin theory of depression: a systematic umbrella review of the evidence', *Molecular Psychiatry*, 20 July 2022, pp. 1–14 <doi.org/10.1038/s41380-022-01661-0>

42. Kirsch, I. et al., 'Initial Severity and Antidepressant Benefits: A Meta-Analysis of Data Submitted to the Food and Drug Administration', *PLoS Medicine*, 26 February 2008, vol. 5 no. 2 <doi.org/10.1371/journal.pmed.0050045>

43. Kelly, K., Posternak, M. & Jonathan, E.A., 'Toward achieving optimal response: understanding and managing antidepressant side effects', *Dialogues in Clinical Neuroscience*, 2008, vol. 10 no. 4, pp. 409–18 <doi.org/10.31887/DCNS.2008.10.4/kkelly>

44. Jureidini, J. & McHenry, L.B., *The Illusion of Evidence-Based Medicine: Exposing the crisis of credibility in clinical research*, Adelaide: Wakefield Press, 2020

45. Moore, J. with Jureidini, J., 'Jon Jureidini – Evidence-Based Medicine in a Post-Truth World', *Mad in America*, 7 September 2022 <madinamerica.com/2022/09/jon-jureidini-evidence-based-medicine-post-truth-world>

46. Hari, J., *Lost Connections*, p. 195

47. Vukasin, F., 29 July 2022, *What doctors think about antidepressants and the 'serotonin theory'*, Royal Australian College of General

Practitioners (RACGP) <www1.
racgp.org.au/newsgp/clinical/
what-doctors-think-about-
antidepressants-and-the-s>

48. van der Kolk, B.A., *The Body Keeps
the Score: Brain, mind, and body
in the healing of trauma*, New
York, NY: Viking, 2014

49. Tripathi, A., Das, A. & Kar, S.K.,
'Biopsychosocial Model in
Contemporary Psychiatry:
Current Validity and Future
Prospects', *Indian Journal
of Psychological Medicine*,
November 2019, vol. 41 no. 6,
pp. 582–5 <doi.org/10.4103/
IJPSYM.IJPSYM_314_19>

50. Merrick, M.T. et al., 'Unpacking
the impact of adverse childhood
experiences on adult mental
health', *Child Abuse & Neglect*,
July 2017, vol. 69, pp. 10–19 <doi.
org/10.1016/j.chiabu.2017.03.016>

51. World Health Organization, 2022,
Social Determinants of Health
<who.int/health-topics/social-
determinants-of-health>

52. Maté, G., *When the Body Says
No: The hidden cost of stress*,
Toronto: Knopf Canada, 2003

53. Egger, J.W., 'Biopsychosocial
Medicine and Health – the
body mind unity theory and its
dynamic definition of health',
Psychologische Medizin, 2015,
vol. 24 no. 1, pp. 24–9 <doi.
org/10.13140/RG.2.1.2334.5361>

54. Mokgobi, M.G., 'Towards
integration of traditional healing
and western healing: Is this
a remote possibility?', *African
Journal for Physical Health
Education, Recreation, and
Dance*, 19 November 2013,
pp. 47–57

55. Vanbuskirk, S., 10 January 2023,
*How Emotions and Organs
Are Connected in Traditional
Chinese Medicine*, Verywell
Mind <verywellmind.com/

emotions-in-traditional-chinese-
medicine-88196>

56. Baikie, K.A. & Wilhelm, K.,
'Emotional and physical
health benefits of expressive
writing', *Advances in Psychiatric
Treatment*, 2005, vol. 11 no. 5,
pp. 338–46 <doi.org/10.1192/
apt.11.5.338>

57. Buck, D. & Ewbank, L., 4
November 2020, *What is social
prescribing?*, The Kings Fund
<kingsfund.org.uk/publications/
social-prescribing>

58. The Big Anxiety, *About*, accessed
1 August 2023 <thebiganxiety.org/
about>

Chapter 3: Human Kind

1. Ross, G., *Inciting Joy: Essays*, Chapel
Hill, NC: Algonquin Books, 2022

2. Dana, D., *The Polyvagal Theory
in Therapy: Engaging the rhythm
of regulation*, New York, NY: W.W.
Norton, 2018

3. Complex Post-Traumatic
Stress Disorder (C-PTSD) is the
experience of ongoing relational
trauma. 'Unlike Post-Traumatic
Stress Disorder (PTSD), Complex
PTSD typically involves being hurt
by another person. These hurts
are ongoing, repeated, and often
involving a betrayal and loss of
safety.' CPTSD Foundation, *What
is CPTSD?*, accessed 14 August
2023 <cptsdfoundation.org/
what-is-complex-post-traumatic-
stress-disorder-cptsd>

4. Ross, G., *Inciting Joy*

5. Collier, S., 17 October 2022, *How
can you find joy (or at least
peace) during difficult times?*,
Harvard Health Publishing
<health.harvard.edu/blog/
how-can-you-find-joy-or-at-
least-peace-during-difficult-
times-202210062826>

6. McKee, L.G. et al., 'Picture This!
Bringing joy into Focus and

Developing Healthy Habits of
Mind: Rationale, design, and
implementation of a randomized
control trial for young adults',
*Contemporary Clinical Trials
Communications*, September
2019, vol. 15 no. 100391 <doi.
org/10.1016/j.conctc.2019.100391>

7. Ward, D., 2023, *In Search of
Duende*, Language Magazine
<languagemagazine.com/in-
search-of-duende>

8. van der Kolk, B.A., *The Body Keeps
the Score: Brain, mind, and body
in the healing of trauma*, New
York, NY: Viking, 2014

9. Bancroft, J.M., *Hoodie Economics:
Changing our systems to value
what matters*, Melbourne: Hardie
Grant, 2023

10. van der Kolk, B.A., *The Body Keeps
the Score*, p. 17

11. Berman, M.G., Jonides, J. &
Kaplan, S., 'The Cognitive Benefits
of Interacting with Nature',
Psychological Science, December
2008, vol. 19 no. 12, pp. 1207–12

12. Williams, D., *Nature, Our
Medicine: How the natural
world sustains us*, Melbourne:
Currawong Books, 2022

13. Wohlleben, P., *The Hidden Life of
Trees: What they feel, how they
communicate – discoveries from
a secret world*, Melbourne: Black
Inc., 2016

14. Ivers, R. & Astell-Burt, T., 'Nature
Rx: Nature prescribing in general
practice', *Australian Journal of
General Practice*, 1 April 2023,
vol. 52 no. 24, pp. 183–7 <doi.org/
10.31128/AJGP-01-23-6671>

15. Huynh, Q. et al., 'Exposure
to public natural space as a
protective factor for emotional
well-being among young people
in Canada', *BMC Public Health*,
29 April 2013, vol. 13 no. 1, pp.
1–14 <doi.org/10.1186/1471-2458-
13-407>

16. German Centre for Integrative Biodiversity Research (iDiv) Halle-Jena-Leipzig, 4 Dec 2020, *Biological diversity evokes happiness* <sciencedaily.com/releases/2020/12/201204110246.htm>

17. Marianne Wobcke, Understanding Country, accessed 1 August 2023 <understandingcountry.com.au/about.html>

18. Yunkaporta, T., *Sand Talk: How Indigenous thinking can save the world*, Melbourne: Text Publishing, 2019

19. Australia Council for the Arts, February–May 2022, *Connected Lives: Creative solutions to the mental health crisis* <australiacouncil.gov.au/advocacy-and-research/arts-creativity-and-mental-wellbeing-policy-development-program>

20. Wohlleben, P., *The Hidden Life of Trees*

21. Dana, D., *Anchored: How to befriend your nervous system using polyvagal theory*, New York, NY: St. Martin's Press, 2022

22. Callaghan, P., *The Dreaming Path: Indigenous thinking to change your life*, Sydney: Bloomsbury, 2022

Chapter 4: Brain Wave

1. The Nap Ministry, *About*, accessed 1 August 2023 <thenapministry.wordpress.com/about>

2. People with Disability Australia, 2023, *Social model of disability* <pwd.org.au/resources/models-of-disability>

3. Siegel, D., *The Developing Mind: How relationships and the brain interact to shape who we are*, New York, NY: The Guilford Press, 1999

4. Mobbs, D. et al., 'The ecology of human fear: survival optimization and the nervous system', *Frontiers in Neuroscience*, 18 March 2015, vol. 9 no. 55 <doi.org/10.3389/fnins.2015.00055>

5. Dana, D., *Befriending Your Nervous System: Looking through the lens of polyvagal theory*, Louisville, CO: Sounds True, 2020

6. Known as 'neurogenic tremors', shaking has been identified by trauma therapists as a highly effective way to release difficult emotions and regulate the nervous system.

7. van der Kolk, B.A., *The Body Keeps the Score: Brain, mind, and body in the healing of trauma*, New York, NY: Viking, 2014, p. 17

8. Porges, S.W., *The Pocket Guide to the Polyvagal Theory: The transformative power of feeling safe*, New York, NY: Norton Professional Books, 2017

9. Eisenberg-Guyot, J. & Prins, S.J., 'The impact of capitalism on mental health: An epidemiological perspective', in Bhugra, D. Moussaoui, D. & Craig, T.J. (eds), *Oxford Textbook of Social Psychiatry*, Oxford: Oxford University Press 2022, pp. 195–204

10. Hersey, T., *Rest is Resistance: A manifesto*, New York, NY: Little Brown Spark, 2022, p. 183

11. Wood, C., 'Reading isn't Shopping', in Wood, C., *The Luminous Solution*, Sydney: Allen & Unwin, 2021, pp. 141–3

12. Maslow, A.H., 'A theory of human motivation', *Psychological Review*, 1943, vol. 50 no. 4, pp. 370–96 <doi.org/10.1037/h0054346>

13. Orme-Johnson, D.W. & Fergusson, L., 'Global impact of the Maharishi Effect from 1974 to 2017: Theory and Research', *Journal of Maharishi Vedic Research Institute*, 2018, vol. 8, pp. 13–79

14. Orme-Johnson, D.W. et al., 'Field-Effects of Consciousness: A Seventeen-Year Study of the Effects of Group Practice of the Transcendental Meditation and TM-Sidhi Programs on Reducing National Stress in the United States', *World Journal of Social Science*, 14 December 2022, vol. 9 no. 2 <doi.org/10.5430/wjss.v9n2p1>

15. National Academies of Sciences, Engineering, and Medicine, *Social Isolation and Loneliness in Older Adults: Opportunities for the health care system*, Washington, DC: The National Academies Press, 2020

16. O'Sullivan, R. et al., 'Impact of the COVID-19 Pandemic on Loneliness and Social Isolation: A Multi-Country Study', *International Journal of Environmental Research and Public Health*, 23 September 2021, vol. 18 no. 19 <doi.org/10.3390/ijerph18199982>

Chapter 5: The Creative Dispensary

1. Thinking about what helps to replenish, restore and reset ourselves can be helped by also thinking about what costs come with some of our habits. Does that wine every night cost me sleep? Does that hard-core exercise plan actually leave me even more exhausted? Instead of labelling these things as good or bad, it can help to think about them in terms of whether they restore us or cost us something.

2. The term 'habit stacking' was coined by S.J Scott. Scott, S.J., *Habit Stacking: 97 small life changes that take five minutes or less*, Scotts Valley, CA: CreateSpace Independent Publishing Platform, 2014

Acknowledgements

Thank you to the wonderful, patient and supportive team at Murdoch Books, especially Alexandra Payne, Jane Morrow, Justine Harding, Sarah Odgers, Julie Mazur Tribe, Jacqui Porter and Lauren Babula. A big thanks to our editor, Clara Ames, for her discerning skill at taming our first drafts.

We are forever heart-filled and grateful to the people who have helped sow the fields of MakeShift work over the past decade. So many, but special mention to those sown into this book, and who've held us along the way: Marcelo Baez, Helena Fox, Melinda Young, Karen Yello, Emma Saunders, Julie Paterson, Sally Ann Conwell, Elana Stone, Kirli Saunders, Linda Kennedy, Nathan Leslie, Angie Cass, Narelle Happ, Nooky, Clare Thackway, Peachy, Mignon Steele and Pete Golsby-Walsh. Gratitude to cherished mentors Monica Davidson, Tanya Van Der Water and Meg West.

For holding us through the writing process, with early draft feedback, advice and playlists, Lizzie Buckmaster Dove and Marianne Wobcke.

Deep thanks to big-hearted generous people who chatted to us, shared themselves and their time for our research: Dr Mark Melek, Dr Mark Baxter, Michele Elliot, Dr Kathryn Boydell, Dr Christina Davies, Helena Norberg-Hodge, Jono Brand, Rebecca Lang, Vanessa Edwige, Dr Paul Callaghan, Dr Annie Werner, Jack Manning Bancroft, Sarah Ball, Charlotte Wood, Carrie Lumby, Liv O'Leary, Megan Goodwin and Mel Cheng.

To every participant, volunteer and staff member of MakeShift in all its iterations. To the brave creative 'inch by inch' of every participant in our ReMind program. We're especially grateful to those who shared their story for this book. And thank you to everyone who kindly gifted us a creative prescription to share, too.

Immense thanks for her incredible illustrations to the inimitable Kiara Mucci, who plucks our vision right out of our heads with such ease, spark and colour.

To Damian, Jemima, Nessie, Ann, Kaija, Colin, Steph and Jedda. Thanks for all the singing.

Find out more about MakeShift at **makeshift.org.au**
Follow us on Instagram at **@makeshift_creative.first.aid**

Caitlin

Deep thanks to Bellambi Lagoon and Woonona rockpools of Dharawal Country, on which my feet travelled miles in crafting and solving the puzzles for this book.

I'm thankful to have spent life so far in the midst of so many curious, sparky friends and inspiring work colleagues. To my faves who make space for my nonsense, and are Here for All of It: Kayte, Edi, Sarah H, Bianca, Cass.

To Lizzie, my comrade and dear friend, who sees me and meets me in work, life and play with such grace, curiosity, deep tender care, and silliness.

For Jamie, Clara and Banjo, my world. You bring glimmers of joy and awe in the mess of life each and every day. I dedicate this book to my dad, who has showed me how to be curious from as far back as I can remember.

Check out fullstop.org.au to donate to this important, incredible service.

Lizzie

The writing of this book coincided with a monumental time in my life. An unexpected outcome of shaping *Creative First Aid* was the roots that it helped to grow and the support it provided. The content I was writing about became a trusty resource. I'm grateful to Dharawal land and its offerings of regular interactions with a solitary pelican, a gentle beckoning to glimpse the sunrise, wild spaces to walk barefoot and seapools to plunge into. To the tallest tree in my local forest, thanks for your wisdom.

A few treasured friends shone bright and held space for me. Special thanks to Annie Walker, Lizzie BD, Annie Werner, Meg W, Emma R, Si and Reine. And to dear Caitlin, thank you for always turning up; not only would this book not even be here without you, but the wide-open ears, occasional challenging nudges, outright hilarity and brain-bursting ideas you offered meant that co-authoring a book alongside you was nothing short of an honour.

Thank you to Marianne B for being so patient with me and listening as I found my voice.

To Nessie and our beloved brown-eyed boys, Harry and Clancy, this book is for you and your courageous creative hearts.

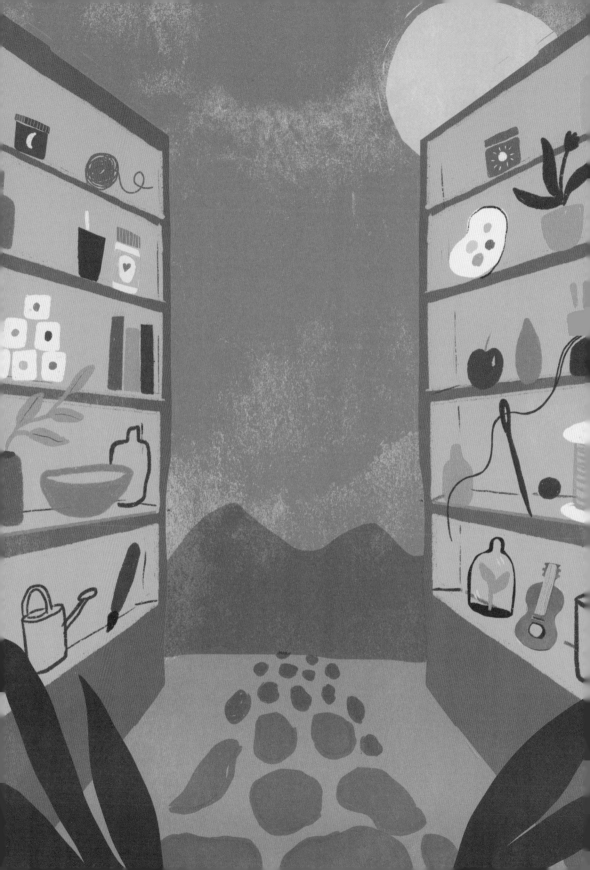

Index

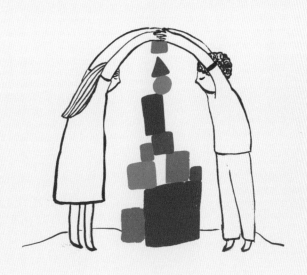

Published in 2024 by Murdoch Books, an imprint of Allen & Unwin

Murdoch Books Australia
Cammeraygal Country
83 Alexander Street
Crows Nest NSW 2065
Phone: +61 (0)2 8425 0100
murdochbooks.com.au
info@murdochbooks.com.au

Murdoch Books UK
Ormond House
26–27 Boswell Street
London WC1N 3JZ
Phone: +44 (0) 20 8785 5995
murdochbooks.co.uk
info@murdochbooks.co.uk

For corporate orders and custom publishing, contact our business development team
at salesenquiries@murdochbooks.com.au

Publisher: Alexandra Payne
Commissioning editor: Julie Mazur Tribe
Editorial manager: Justine Harding
Design manager: Sarah Odgers
Designers: Northwood Green, Lauren Babula
Editor: Clara Ames
Illustrator: Kiara Mucci
Production director: Lou Playfair

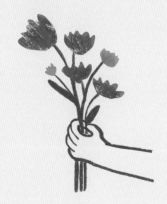

*Murdoch Books acknowledges the Traditional Owners
of the Country on which we live and work. We pay our
respects to all Aboriginal and Torres Strait Islander
Elders, past and present.*

ISBN 978 1 92261 683 8

 A catalogue record for this
book is available from the
National Library of Australia

A catalogue record for this book is available from the
British Library

Printed by C&C Offset Printing Co. Ltd., China

10 9 8 7 6 5 4 3 2 1

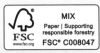
FSC
www.fsc.org
MIX
Paper | Supporting
responsible forestry
FSC® C008047

Caitlin Marshall and **Lizzie Rose** are the founders
of MakeShift, an award-winning agency that provides
trauma-informed creativity and mental health programs
for communities, workplaces and groups throughout
Australia. Since 2013 they have worked with thousands
of people, including first responders; communities
affected by bushfires and floods; corporate clients such
as Atlassian, Kimberly-Clark and Ikea; and organisations
including ABC TV, Sydney Opera House, Support Act,
NSW Department of Juvenile Justice, Creative Australia
and Black Dog Institute. Caitlin is also a qualified social
worker and trainer in vicarious trauma management
and gender-based violence who has had one foot in the
creative arts since adolescence. Lizzie is a community
development practitioner, sustainability educator and
qualified yoga teacher. Find them at makeshift.org.au
or on Instagram at @makeshift_creative.first.aid.